THE
QUIET
VET

INTO THE SUNSET

CW01433022

The Quiet Vet... Into The Sunset

Copyright © Rod Wood 2023 All Rights Reserved

The rights of Rod Wood to be identified as the author of this work have been asserted in accordance with the Copyright, Designs and Patents Act 1988

All rights reserved. No part may be reproduced, adapted, stored in a retrieval system or transmitted by any means, electronic, mechanical, photocopying, or otherwise without the prior written permission of the author or publisher.

Book Printing UK
Remus House
Coltsfoot Drive
Woodston
Peterborough
PE2 9BF

www.bookprintinguk.com

A CIP catalogue record for this book is available from the British Library.

The views expressed in this work are solely those of the author and do not necessarily reflect the views of the publisher, and the publisher hereby disclaims any responsibility for them

ISBN: 978-1-3999-5739-7

THE QUIET VET

INTO THE SUNSET

ROD WOOD

BookPrintingUK
Peterborough
2023

Other Books by Rod Wood

Kilimanjaro. My Goal. My Story.

(republished as Kilimanjaro. My Story)

Fishing the Net. (with Jane Reeves).

Kenya. A Mountain to Climb.

The Quiet Vet.

*Dedicated to Jane and Jill for their
continued support in these projects*

Contents

Author's Biography

*S*INCE *MY EARLY teens I had decided on a veterinary career and qualified from Bristol University in 1977. That was the start of a career spanning forty five years until I retired 1n 2022.*

I am a dairy farmer's son so my interest was always in farm practice, and that has been my main speciality throughout my career, mainly in the South-West and Shropshire. I have always loved the outdoors and the countryside. There have been the odd dabbles at small animal work, but for the last seventeen years of my career I have had the pleasure of working solely on farm.

It has been a career with its ups and downs, including working through two epidemics, and experiencing the affects this can have on ones well-being. But throughout, it has been a pleasure to be involved with the farming community, and offer what help I can.

Married twice and with two children, now well grown-up, but neither of whom wanted to follow in father's footsteps. Jane and I will now pursue our interests in retirement but hopefully nearer the coast where I can indulge in my walking, gardening and hopefully golf again. In the later part of my life, I have found that I enjoy writing, especially on East Africa, an area I have been privileged to visit on three occasions so far, but is certainly on my wish list to return again, maybe even to climb one of its mountains again.

A largely happy career that I hope I may have conveyed in this book, along with the changing times in farm practice.

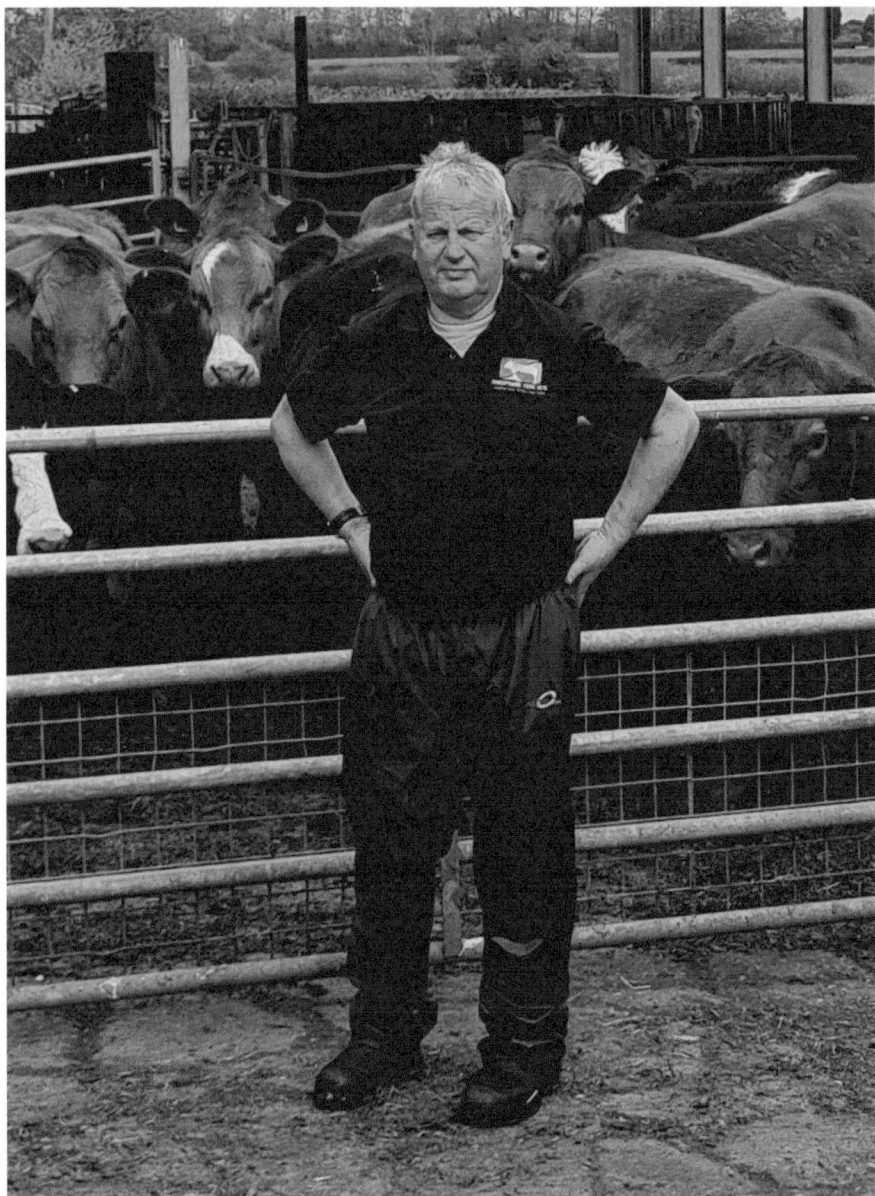

Early One Morning:

Early Summer, 1978.

OR SHOULD THIS chapter be named the prologue; I must start somewhere?

Life had taken me to Cullopmton in East Devon, and I had settled into a practice much to my liking, a predominately farm animal practice with some horse and small animal work. But I was green, I had my farming background to call on and had some great tutors on the way through my training at university, but, and it was a big but, I was only out of university a few months and it was now time to show my worth. Eventually, I would have to stand on my own two feet and cope with whatever was thrown at me.

Here I was at last having to deal with my first weekend on call in my new practice and expected to deal with such emergencies that come my way.

My short stay in Buckinghamshire, I had done my duties, but it was rare to get a call "out of hours." Now I was working in a busy farm animal practice and let us be honest, a cow does not know whether it is Wednesday, Friday, or Sunday, or do they! A sick cow is a sick cow whatever time of day it is and whatever day it might be. I had done nights on call while I was in Devon but now it was time to do my first weekend.

The rota worked that if you were on call for the weekend then us assistants would be on first call on Friday night, and this particular one had passed reasonably peacefully for me. Anything less than three evening calls would be classed as quiet, so Friday had been quiet. Four of us would work until Saturday lunchtime, then for the rest of the weekend there would be two of us, me working with the senior partner in my early days. He would be on first call from Saturday lunchtime until nine o'clock Sunday morning then we would swop over, me on first, him on second call though his wife would have the phones to take calls and pass them onto me, or him if necessary if I got too inundated.

What would be a quiet weekend? I did not know but was about to find out, this was going to be my first in East Devon in an intensive cattle practice. I was about to gain my first experience of a farm practice weekend. Saturday had been quiet, other than a couple of calls in the morning and of course as I had soon learnt in this practice, if you got called out to something, there would almost certainly be a lame cow or four while "you'm here!" A peaceful afternoon though as I lived above the office and there was no such thing as a mobile phone in those days, I was basically confined to barracks. But to be honest, I did not know anyone in the area so wouldn't be painting the town red on Saturday night.

Sunday would come round soon enough. I had the thought wondering if Oliver would wait on any early calls until we had swopped over so I would be doing them, or would he do the honourable thing and do them himself. My commencement time for being first on call duly passed and it was not long before my phone rang, and I was informed of my first call.

A cow with what the farmer said was Milk Fever, and the joy of working in this practice was that almost all calls would be close to practice base. If I had to drive more than fifteen miles, it was a long journey. We had many dairy clients, but being an intensive dairy area, they were all close to each other, calls would often be to next door. This call was no more than three miles away, I would be there in no time at all, out of town, a drive down a back road and I would be there, and I had been there before so it would not be a stranger visiting this "emergency". I had seen plenty of cases of Milk Fever when growing up on Dad's farm, the characteristic cow straight after calving who could not stand up, would be lying down in sternal recumbency and with an S bend kink in her neck. Even in my embryonic career I knew that if a farmer said it was Milk Fever, then that is what it was likely to be, and one should get on and treat the cow straight away.

I arrived on the farm and collecting my things I followed the farmer into the field where said cow was lying, with her kinked neck and her newly born calf lying near by waiting patiently for mum to stand up so it could get a drink of milk from her. One hoped that the calf had managed to get sufficient colostrum from mum to get all those necessary antibodies in her first milk which would ensure a healthy start to its life.

The symptoms of Milk Fever are largely determined by the levels of Magnesium in the cow's blood, despite it being a hypocalcaemia, low levels of Calcium in the blood stream which causes a generalised muscular weakness. If just Calcium is involved then you will see the cow that I have described above, lying there but too weak to stand up. If she is low in Magnesium as well then more often than not, she would be lying flat out on her side often with her legs paddling, signs of grass staggers, grass tetany.

As in this case where the cow is in a field, then it is often not possible to get the car to the cow so unless a long way away when the farmer would take you to the cow in his Land Rover or tractor, you walked and would have to carry all you thought you may need to treat the cow.

A halter to restrain her with, though she was lying down, it would be beneficial to turn her head to one side to find her jugular vein. A "flutter valve", rubber tubing with a needle attachment one end and on the other a valve which attached to a bottle that the drug would be administered through with an air bleed in it to let air into the bottle while the fluid went into the cow. A needle of course, of a suitable wide bore to allow a steady infusion of the fluid into the cow, then the standard stuff you needed to examine a cow, thermometer, stethoscope, rectal glove, and lube and probably some uterine pessaries. Then of course there would be the drugs. In those days, Calcium came in brown four hundred ml. glass bottles. They were nice colour coded with different coloured tops, green for 40% straight Calcium Borogluconate, red would be 20% Calcium with Phosphorus in it, blue would be 20% Calcium with both Phosphorus and Magnesium added, black straight Magnesium Sulphate and gold would be 40% Glucose. It made it easy to pick which bottles you wanted out of a case in the boot of the car, even in relative darkness. But I had decided that for the sake of ease that I would use a green top and a blue top in most cases, rather than carrying a complete selection with me to every case.

I had loaded my necessary equipment into pockets in my coat and set off across the field with the farmer towards the stricken cow. He was convinced the cow had Milk Fever and expected me to start treatment straight away, and glancing at her I had no reason to think any differently. We would soon find my expertise (or not) at finding a vein in a cow.

The halter was placed over the cow's head, something she resented and did try and make a feeble attempt to stand up, but flopped back down again before the farmer pulled her head around to one side leaving me the other side to find her jugular vein. Somewhere in our training we had been told by an instructor to put a string or thin rope around her neck to try and raise the vein, bending her neck around often making the vein stand out quite obviously. Then one would push the needle through the skin over the vein and direct it through and up the vein, noting a flow of blood out of the needle. A good flow of deep red blood then one was in the vein, a gushing of bright red blood meant one had gone to deep and had found the carotid artery transporting blood up to the head and brain. This was a high-pressure blood vessel and there was no way Calcium would flow through the flutter valve into it. More likely was that the flow would be the other way and the bottle would start filling with blood.

Well here goes, it was time for me to demonstrate my "skills". I did try the string round the neck thing, baler twine was plentiful in those days, "farmers friend" as it was often called, as it served so many different purposes. A vein in sight, I inserted my needle through the skin then into the vein. Success first time as venous blood flowed out so all I needed to do now was to attach the flutter valve with bottle on, a green top, and let the Calcium go slowly into the vein, the blood stream to correct this cow's deficiency. As it entered the cow, air flowed through the valve into the bottle which I held up in the air allowing it to empty slowly into the cow. I knew that one could not give the Calcium too fast, it may have dire consequences on the heart if I did, I did not want to kill the cow while trying to save her and the farmer would not be impressed. Over a few minutes the bottle emptied into the cow's vein, but even during those few minutes I was finding that even such a light weight got heavy as I held the bottle up in the air, my arms were feeling tired. More so when that bottle was emptied and I then had to remove the needle from the vein and replace it under the skin of the cow just behind her shoulder, in the loose skin over her rib cage and then give another 400ml., a blue top this time, again holding the bottle up while it slowly emptied. Finally, it was done, the cow had received two bottles of Calcium, one intravenously, the other subcutaneously.

I then checked her over, getting the farmer to lift a back leg up so I could look at her udder and make sure there were no signs of mastitis. The calf got quite excited as I expressed some milk to check it was okay, breakfast at last the calf thought! A listen to her chest, check her temperature, check her internally per vagina to make sure there was not another calf and to see if she had passed her afterbirth and I was finished.

All I needed to do now was to give her a nudge in her ribs and hopefully she would stand up. She did, my first case had concluded well, and calf was now pleased to see mum standing so it could feed. But we must not let it have too much to start with otherwise mum's Calcium reserves would be depleted quickly.

I collected my equipment together, went back to the farm buildings to wash off and then back into the car, it was time to go.

But a message had been left at the farmhouse, I had another call to go to, and you guessed it, another cow with Milk Fever but luckily for me it was not far away but did sound a bit more urgent.

I was on my way, soon arriving at the next farm, putting on my boots, loading my coat again with a bottle in each pocket, the other necessary things I needed and set off across another field with the farmer to see my next victim. This cow was obviously in more distress than my first case of the day, she was flat out on her side, quite distressed and not being able to eructate, burp, she was starting to get a bit blown. The gas could not escape from her rumen which was starting to distend. In extremise this would put pressure on her diaphragm making breathing harder and there was a risk that she could regurgitate and then inhale some of her rumen contents.

No time to lose, she needed Calcium and probably Magnesium as well to be administered into her as soon as possible. But she was distressed so was fighting us, but we managed to extend her head and neck forward which made seeing the jugular vein easy, it standing engorged in its groove along the bottom of the neck. No need for "farmer's friend" here, it was standing out ready to have a needle put in it and the flow of blood out soon followed. We would have to be careful again not to give the Calcium too quickly and I would also give some of the blue top containing Magnesium into the vein as well so her Mag reserves would rise quicker.

But of course, I was holding bottles up in the air again as they slowly emptied through the flutter valve into the blood stream, and although they should be getting lighter as they emptied, they certainly did not feel like it. Swopping the bottle from hand to hand only meant that both arms were beginning to feel just as tired as each other. But at last, both were empty and with a little effort the farmer and I managed to get the cow sitting up properly on her sternum.

It is surprising how quickly these cows will respond. She sat up and immediately there was a large burp as she managed to release some of the gas from her rumen which now visibly deflated in front of our eyes. As the Calcium worked, her muscles started to work again, and she immediately peed as her bladder muscles kicked into action. How she needed to empty that! From a cow that looked desperate, she now was alert, looking for her calf and making vague attempts to get to her feet. I completed my examination of her and could not find anything else untoward. We tidied up around her before again that gentle nudge which would bring her to her feet. It worked, the cow was happy, the farmer was happy, and I was happy as we had reached a satisfactory conclusion to the case. She staggered uneasily for a few paces before spreading her four pins out wide to steady her balance and after five minutes one would not have known there had been anything wrong with her.

It was time to go back to the buildings and again wash off ready to see if there were any more calls. There was and it looked like I was going to get plenty of practice today as it was yet another case of Milk Fever, but again not far away. I would have a quick chance to catch my breath before going through the same procedure again at a different place. But even this early in my career I was getting to refine my methods.

With all this equipment to carry each time, and the farmer was keen that the Calcium bottles should be warmed up so that they would be as near to body temperature when infused into the cow rather than the temperature they were in when in the boot of my car, a bucket of hot water was provided that I could put the bottles in to transport them to the cow, along with the flutter valve and needle. This allowed the rest to go into my coat pockets, and even if the time taken to reach the cow was not sufficient to have made that much difference to the temperature of the bottles sitting in the bucket, the farmer was happy it was warmer and it had made carrying easier.

It also provided me with something to wash with as after successfully inserted the needle into the vein, my hands would invariably be covered in blood. But of course, there was nothing that got me out of holding those damn bottles up in the air again as their contents slowly went into the cow. The subcutaneous injection would leave a swelling and I tried to massage this, disperse the liquid under the skin while it was going in, one arm in the air holding the bottle, the other pressing gently on this swelling, but this was a little uncomfortable for the cow. Another successful conclusion and my confidence was rising, three successful attempts at inserting this huge needle into a vein and at the end of it, three cows standing up soon afterwards. Everyone happy except for my aching arms. And if the farmer had carried the full bucket of water and bottles across the field to the cow, then when I had finished, we could empty it for a lighter journey back.

It must be time for a cup of coffee, and as it was lucky I was living in a flat over the office I was soon home, and over that much needed cup I reloaded the car with a fast depleting stock of Calcium bottles in my boot. It was a chance to also wash through my flutter valve which was getting so much use already that day. If you do not wash them out thoroughly then with the forty percent Calcium, it can start crystallising out in the narrower parts and cause a blockage. So many times, later in my career that I would find this an utter inconvenience and would have to unblock it somehow or another, hot water usually did the trick (another advantage of carrying the bottles and flutter valve to the cow in a bucket of hot water!).

On this first Sunday on call, it would not be long before I would be wanted again, and surprise, surprise it was for another Milk Fever, and then another and then another. Nine in total I did that day, and just for variety I did no other calls other than Milk Fevers. And just for good measure as my duty finished at eight on the Monday morning, I did two more before my normal day started when the office officially opened. As the Sunday progressed it was obvious how tired my arm was getting as the bottles I were holding got held lower and lower, and I would swop from arm to arm ever more frequently. When it was time for my bed, it was more than welcome. A terribly busy day for my first weekend duty, it would be a long while until I had another that had been so busy. And certainly, I never in my whole career had another Milk Fever day as I did then, I can remember one Sunday when I did eleven lambings but that day I did see a couple of other things and finished off with a cow caesarean just for a bit of variety. The wonderful thing was that all those cases of Milk Fever responded so quickly and there was not one of them that was not standing when I left the farm. Very satisfying and I had successfully found the vein in every case, and it was only the first one that I used the string and have not used one since.

I did often wonder why on a spring morning with a heavy dew why cases were more prevalent, compared with dry mornings or even when it was wet. Did other minerals such as Potassium, high in spring, inhibit Calcium and Magnesium uptake? Did I ever produce an answer, no, I do not think I did! Devon in those days forty plus years ago was a big dairy area producing a lot of milk off grass. Therefore, there were many cows that calved in the spring to coincide with maximum grass production. It was our busiest time of year, those months from March through to the end of May, holidays taken at that time were frowned upon as we would be too busy to cope with reduced staff. We would be overrun with the likes of Milk Fevers, calvings and caesareans, cows with Grass Staggers, displaced abomasums and of course it was lambing time as well.

But in those days, unlike today, farmers were unwilling to try treating cases of Milk Fever themselves. They may put a bottle of Calcium under the skin but would never try having a go at the vein, even in extreme emergency.

Milk fever is a disease primarily of dairy cattle though it is seen occasionally in beef and other species. Also called parturient paresis or post parturient hypocalcaemia, it is caused by reduced calcium levels in the bloodstream. This infers that it is normally seen after a cow has calved, but it can occur before calving and may delay the onset of calving because of the affect it has on stopping muscle contractions of the uterus.

Cows are dried off, stopped being milked, a few weeks before their next calf is due to give them time to recover from their lactation while the calf is growing rapidly inside her. The cow's dietary needs are reduced, as is her need for Calcium as she is not producing milk. When she calves there is a sudden demand for calcium for colostrum and then milk production and that demand exceeds the body's ability to mobilise calcium into the bloodstream. So more often than not, it is not so much a deficiency but a lack of ability to get it where it is needed, from the bones into milk. There is some hormonal control involved in this and it is more common in older cows whose milk yield will tend to be higher. Also, there is a higher incidence in Channel Island breeds, the Jersey and Guernsey.

A weekend of success in treating what was then, forty years ago a very common condition, called a fever though in almost all cases there is no elevation in body temperature. With the warning that if Calcium is given into the vein too quickly causing it to stop the heart, treatment was then always invariably successful, injecting the cow, waiting a short while then with a little encouragement she would rise to her feet. I had seen it in dad's cows, but even if he was somewhat of a pioneer in farming techniques, using steaming up rations to prepare the cow from the change from her dry period to that of milk production, I don't think the phrase "transition cow management" had been invented then, he did lose the best cow he ever had with Milk Fever. A cow by the lovely name of Spindleberry calved successfully, but on returning into the herd and despite regular observation, her milk production caused such demands on her reserves of calcium that she went down in the cubicles and got herself into a position where she could not right herself. Her rumen filled with gas, put too much pressure on her chest, her heart and she was lost, she would die. A cow that would give eleven, twelve gallons of milk a day, a big loss.

Milk fever has been recorded in veterinary literature since 1793, a long time ago. One heard of such remedies as early as the beginning of the twentieth century, 1901, where the udder would be inflated with air and this was reportedly a successful treatment as long as you didn't give the cow mastitis while doing this, i.e., hygiene was essential.

We did of course move on and the introduction of injectable forms of Calcium were highly successful in treating this condition. But as I was to learn, other factors then started to be implicated in our differential diagnosis of seeing a "Downer" cow. Many of those early cases in my career responded but then we started to find a few that did not, perhaps not typical of the disease where cows just wouldn't get up, none of the S-bend in their neck, they just sat there and looked at you. We would soon find out about the role of Vitamin E and Selenium in cows and areas like where I was in Devon, we would learn this was a deficient area. Cows which had injured themselves, slipping and damaging nerves, muscles, and even breaking limbs. Cows which at calving, especially in dirty conditions would develop mastitis, an inflammation of the udder caused by invading bacteria, some of these would turn toxic, making the cow seriously ill and before the advent of fluid therapy in cattle, invariably fatal.

Cases of "Downer" cows were becoming more complex and over time I did not see the immediate response to treatment that I got on that first Sunday. The wonderful ways some farmers had of trying to persuade a cow to stand after treatment, pouring water down her ear or getting the faithful farm dog to jump on the cow's back and bark in an attempt to get her out of her slumber! Some cases obviously needed urgent infusion of Calcium if flat out, and their response would be an aid to diagnosis, but a more thorough examination of some cases would often be needed to find some other or some concurrent disease.

But as my career progressed, even those straightforward cases seemed to take longer to respond. The times of giving her a shove and she got up seemed less common and one would have to prop the cow up with straw bales (alas now also a rare commodity) so she could stay sitting up until she was ready to stand, whether it be a couple of hours later or up to a couple of days, and one may have to make the decision whether she would ever stand again, the longer she lay, the more muscle damage that could occur. Over the course of time, cows could receive four, five, ten bottles of

Calcium plus other drugs that may help her, anti-inflammatories when they became available, corticosteroids in my early days and stimulants such as Vetibenzamine, another of those drugs that seemed to work but is no longer available.

The nature of intensive dairy farming was changing, the breeds were changing to large high production Holsteins and with that the management of these milk factories had to change as well. We still saw the old-fashioned Milk Fevers in traditional low production herds milking their cows off grass, but these high yielding cows spent more and more time housed so their feeding, their diet could be managed more scientifically.

A call would come in late at night or early in the morning and it would still be for a cow down with milk fever, but when I arrived on the farm I wouldn't be led across a field to find the cow but into a dark shed, if you were lucky into a calving box with lights, but no, into this dark shed with mounds of straw, manure, other cows lying about in the dark trying to get their forty winks only to be disturbed by veterinary clambering around by torchlight trying to find the afflicted cow. We would still probably get our bucket of hot, or more likely tepid water to warm our bottles of Calcium, and a quick observation of the cow would decide whether to get the Calcium into the cow as quickly as possible or whether to look for other disease signs that may be present dictating a different course of action. The halter was still a necessity, and then perching your torch somewhere where it could highlight the cow's neck, her jugular, I would place my large needle into the vein and administer the Calcium, then the rest subcutaneously. What a blessing it was when these head torches were invented so you could direct your light always where you wanted, like towards the vein in the neck!

But of course by this time, all those cows deep in slumber were now aroused, not only by a light and a vet to come and lick, sniff, bunt, but also a bucket which if it did contain water and bottles of Calcium, may, just may contain some nuts or some corn which they were only to keen to eat. How many times when holding up those bottles did some cow stick her nose into the bucket and pull it over, spilling all my water. When done I would walk back to the car, my hands covered with blood from being unable to wash them after finding the vein with the blood pouring out over them before I attached the flutter valve to the needle.

And of course, by now, that little prod when you had finished, cows did not get up in this modern era, milk fever had become a far more complicated problem.

And the days of getting those little bales to push in behind the cow's shoulder and by her hip bones, they were gone now too. We now have enormous half tonne bales which need a tractor and fore loader to get in place and you support the cow as best you can with this block. And put there to support the downer cow, there would be plenty of her mates who saw it as food or as a punch bag that they could jostle with in the dark, at least they were using the bale and not me!

Those checks to make sure there are no other problems is still essential, no toxic mastitis, no damaged bones, or damaged nerves in calving. And of course one would have to check that there was not still another calf inside the cow, having injected her, on more than one occasion I would then have to remove another calf from mum, and if she wasn't fed up enough of the sight of one calf trying to chivvy her into action, the sight of another, well! In fairness, once mum had received her Calcium, she was only too happy to exercise her motherly instincts and start to lick and cajole her calves, often being the stimulus to get her back on her feet.

We have taught farmers over the years to be able to treat their own Milk fevers, many do, some are still only happy to inject some Calcium under the skin. Technology, understanding of the disease has moved on, as has management of cows with high yielding Holsteins kept inside at this stage of their cycle with far more dietary management. Complicated calculations can be made balancing the anion/ cation content of their diet so that minerals can be added to diets to correct any imbalances. It would be too much to go into DCAB calculations or even what it means here to describe how diet formulations are reached. But the great unknown is always grass, and for those cows that still go out especially in spring to graze we still rely on tried and trusted old methods of control, and treatment when necessary, and these are the cows that still respond like they did in the "good old "days.

It has been found that oral Calcium gives a better control than subcutaneous Calcium, there now being various boluses or drenches that you can give to help control Milk fever, and for me personally, I always enjoyed giving one of the drenches as to make it more palatable, it was flavoured with aniseed. Whether the cow liked it or not, I just loved the smell of aniseed while I was giving it.

Times change, cows do not respond like they used to, so we now have various bits of equipment to help the cow to her feet, is this physiotherapy of some sort, maybe. At least if we can get her to us her legs, to support her weight for a little while it will encourage her muscle to work and there is often a better outcome if she will not rise herself. The old Bagshaw hoist and the less said about that the better, configurations of straps that worked well once you had figured how they all, worked and where they went. A wonderful inflatable rubber bag that you placed under the cow, then pumped up. In my experience it worked well if the cow was the right size for the support, but if too long or too short how frustrating it was to manoeuvre the cow onto the thing then pump it up only to find the cow falling off the front or the back of it. I am sure the cow lost confidence as well.

Over those forty plus years, how many cows with Milk fever have I treated, hundreds and hundreds and hundreds. How many bottles of Calcium have I held up in the air, double that although the glass bottles were replaced by plastic ones, still fitting the same old flutter valve. Good boy, I always took them to recycling! Many successful cases, some that needed repeat treatments, some that finished off with twenty odd bottles, the farmer would keep on giving them, almost certainly switching off the hormonal control system forever. Cows that I have had to treat and then calve them, others, more often treating post-calving but then having to remove a twin.

If more recently it became at times a frustrating problem to treat, in those early days it was always satisfying to treat, give a nudge and a successful outcome as the cow got to her feet. That in the farmer's eyes always made you look good; you had treated the problem with a positive outcome.

Over time my arms got stronger, I even developed biceps, and I may have refined my techniques a little. But what did experience tell me in the end, or teach me?

When the farmer asked if he could do anything to help.......

"Yes, hold the bloody bottle up for me"!

I could find something else to do to make me look busy but was not so tiring.

LAZY DAYS:

July 2022.

I<small>T HAS BEEN</small> just over thirteen months since I walked out of the door of my workplace for the last time, well not strictly true as because of Covid, our work protocol had meant for the last few months, over a year, we vets in the practice had been working from home. We used the office as a base to pick up drugs and any equipment we may need for our daily chores and did have one room that we could use but strictly on the basis that only four of us could be in there at any one time, socially distancing of course.

Retirement had at last arrived, if a little later than first planned when my career had begun. That final day, sad in so many ways but a relief in others that at last I had committed myself to wind down, a chance now for me to enjoy what I wanted to do when I wanted to and while I was still able to. The sadness was that because of Covid, my leaving my workplace of the past sixteen/seventeen years had not happened as I had hoped. I drove out of the office one final time, risking the dangerous right turn out towards Shrewsbury, that was it, my retirement. But I had not had the chance to say my goodbyes, my farewells to many of my work colleagues, some of the vets I had worked for over the previous few years. Even more disappointing was not being able to say adieu to the farmers that I had served over that time, those which I had built a strong relationship with in a more informal way than just driving off from their farms one last time.

In giving in my notice all those months previously, I had hoped that there would be some sort of leaving do, giving me a chance to say my goodbyes to all. But Covid came along and no "social mixing," there would be no party, not in the immediate future anyway.

"One day," I was told, "We will have a leaving do for you." But when, and if it were too long after I had left, would it mean the same?

I would have to wait and see, but in the meantime, I WAS RETIRED. My life was now my own to spend my time as I pleased and with more time to spend with Jane, my wife now of coming up to four years. Time to explore our world that we live in and to pursue those interests of mine which I had so neglected over the past years.

Retirement day was a Friday, so having given up doing on-calls about eight months previously, there was a weekend to look forward to and on Monday I would not be going to work!

A weekend in Bala with one of my best mates and then it was down to my beloved Dorset with Jane for a few days. Malta had been the plan but with all the uncertainty with flights over Covid, we weren't prepared to take the risk of booking a cruise from Valetta around Italy to return to the island and spend a few days, only to find that it could all be cancelled again like it had when we had planned to do this the previous year. Dorset it would be, returning to a cottage we had stayed in previously in the beautiful village of Symmondsbury. Here we would learn to relax without the thought of having to go back to work after a few days, a new experience for me.

A mixture of walking, meeting friends, idling on beaches, spending a little time with my son, staying in the area but not travelling far and seeing what retirement would be like without the worries of work.

And they were relaxing days as we enjoyed the sunshine of early summer, gentle sea breezes, watching the sunsets from the top of Colmer Hill, a steep but short climb from behind "Cosy Nest", and the multitude of butterflies so serene and gentle busying themselves in this quiet environment. If people say their population is in decline, I have marvelled at the different species and their numbers as they caress the winds and flora around me as I have wandered the more permanent grasslands near the Dorset coast. Enjoyable meals out in the local hostelries, enjoying local bands playing and one memorable night doing a pub quiz when an inspired guess on the last question of the night, a fifty-point answer took us from last to second place.

But of course, there is always a time to come home and face the reality of the real world whatever that may be for be from now on for me. Retirement at last, the time you had worked for through all those years. My time was now my own but how would I adjust to that, the absence of a daily routine which is what work had given me.

I could not, would not completely turn my back on what had been a long career, I had been asked by one or two people if I could help them when I could, and I was pleased to do that as long as they accepted that I only had limited equipment now and certainly no drugs. But if I could give helpful advice, do a little advisory work and the odd bit of real vetting, then I was only too happy to help as long as I would not be treading on the toes of my former employers. I had worked a life with cows, and it would be hard for me to not do anything with them again.

I had been asked if I was willing to go back from time to time to help out if necessary, something I said I could if available but what form that would take, I could only wait and see. More likely than not it would be involve Tuberculosis testing. But that now would be for another day, I had other things in my life to now plan out.

Exploring North Wales further, would we move there at some stage? An invite to the VIP stands at the Tour of Britain cycle race when in Llandudno, walking and climbing in the lakes again and a trip to Mallorca with Jane in October to visit her sister. Most exciting was my son's wedding coming up towards the end of the year, and his stag weekend if I did not consider myself too old to be there, gone were my days of drinking to excess, but perhaps an old head would steady the ship if necessary.

So exciting times to look forward to in retirement. But also unfinished business. I had always said I would never write a vet book, well let's be honest, I had always hated writing until my conquest of Kilimanjaro and with it, overcoming depression. But having wanted to make a permanent history of it if only for myself, I had authored a book on it and others since. *The Quiet Vet* was my initial retirement project, to finish writing it and then to get it published. I had wanted to convey through my experiences as a farm vet how times had changed over my nearly fifty years involved in the profession. Obviously, as in anything, things move on, and mostly for the better but I wanted to highlight those improvements. The change in drugs available, mostly for the better. Now the availability of so many different and effective vaccines, making disease control better. Husbandry changes, better technology making our job easier and better for our patients. Improved surgical techniques, better equipment for handling animals making our and our helpers' jobs safer. But I also wanted to highlight some of the sadness involved in our day to day lives, the affects the whole package can have on our mental health and wellbeing, how like me so many others involved in the profession have suffered over the years and in the past often alone.

But I also wanted to show how some of our food production is carried out, what is involved and the people behind it. Essentially, as farm vets, we are servicing part of the food production of this country, the livestock industry, farming in general, what is the aim of it all? To produce food for the nation, or as much as we can economically. I feel it is important that the general public should understand where the food on their table comes from, how it is produced and by whom, the farmers. Something about their lives, the stresses and toil that they go through, the good times and some of their hardships.

As I say, we as farm vets are part of that industry although we will also serve those smallholders, those people who may just want to keep a few animals for pleasure. The Good Life!

It is a life I have enjoyed, a life that I will still have some contact with and a life that although now retired, I can try and show and give some understanding of what is involved in a profession that I have been involved in from both sides, as a farmer's son and as a farm vet.

Perhaps the characters that I have come across on the way are not as, what's the best way to describe them, rustic, rough, abrasive as those farmers that James Herriot describes from the Yorkshire Dales, but those that I have been involved in all have had their own characters, their own ways and have been special to me in how my career has progressed. They all have their own stories, their own unique ways of doing things, have their own hardships. But all these farmers wherever they have come from are all involved in the same industry, the one that us farm vets are aligned to, and that is producing food for the tables of this land.

But my career has taken me elsewhere, to Africa, somewhere very dear to me. It has involved me in charities, fund raising, and it has involved me in sport.

Being a farm vet has been my life up to this junction where I may take other directions and it would be my wish to share more of my experiences with you, the public. That love of animals, working with cows especially, the rewards and heartaches that have occurred on the way, and perhaps I would just write a little about what I consider to be important issues that don't seem to occupy enough thought by those people who try and run our wonderful country.

So where is a good place to restart my story, getting up and relating just another day at work....

A Day in the Life:

"I READ THE news today, oh boy.
About a lucky man who made the grade"

My alarm was set as usual for six thirty in the morning, another day at work is about to begin. Did I make the grade, well, all those years ago I passed my exams and qualified as a veterinary surgeon. Now, with years of experience and specialising in the part of the job I always wanted to be involved in, namely in farm animal practice, my daily routine was about to begin again in my chosen profession, doing what enjoy most, working in the countryside.

A day in my life, my life as a farm vet. In those early days forty years ago, then my day was somewhat different from the days when I was near the end of my career. Yes, the six thirty alarm was the same, and then breakfast but when my working day began then it was altogether different. I guess that was for two reasons, firstly all those years ago I was a green, new graduate who had picked up some experience when helping dad on the farm when growing up but essentially was still a new vet, and in those days then we did do far more fire brigade work, a lot of which we have now taught farmers to do through many agricultural training courses.

My early days would be spent doing mainly that fire brigade work, the calls that would come in early that day which would then be passed on to especially us youngsters. We had to get on with it, gaining our experience on the hoof, rather than the soft entry the modern new graduate has, when even after qualifying he or she will accompany a more senior vet, seeing what they do and slowly under supervision would have the chance to have a go themselves.

From my first day I was on my own, given a list of calls to do and setting off if a little apprehensively, to do them until all completed by which time, I may have gained a few more. That Sunday with all those milk fevers was a more than busy day for a first weekend on call, and was more than a little nerve racking, but the experience I gained in the long term would have been immense, and the confidence in myself in achieving such positive outcomes. And of course, if the results had been positive, that farmer soon recognised you and greeted you the next time knowing last time turned out fine.

Those early days in Devon where I went from one farm to the next, and then to the next door one as well, intense work, often repetitive especially in the giving of S19 vaccinations to calves to give them some immunity against Brucellosis, and the half dozen lame cows that then followed. But it was a great grounding for a new graduate, a chance to gain a lot of experience in a short length of time and across a broad spectrum of work. Yes, the routine as described above, but also thrown in with that were all the calvings, lambings etc that came in as emergencies because we youngsters were often the most easily available to go on the call, the experienced vets would be on routine farm visits, doing regular and advisory work on their farms on a regular basis and at a set time. These were the calls that would be booked in weeks in advance, happening weekly, fortnightly, or even monthly depending on the individual farmer's needs, but he would usually have the same vet for each visit unless that vet was on holiday. Now we would take a youngster with us on such visits, so they could follow us in examining cows, gaining experience in what they were doing, routine fertility work. Teaching goes on even after graduation.

We learnt the hard way, finding out for ourselves and I guess that for me, that was the best way to learn, get out and do it myself. Those were great days down in Devon back in the late seventies, early eighties and gave me a thorough grounding of what one needed to know and be able to do as a competent farm vet. Long days with lots of different calls (but that lame cow would usually appear whatever you had been called out for in the first place), and somewhere along the line you would find time to write your work up and book it so the accounts department could do the monthly billing. The longer you took to do this, the more likely you were to forget to charge for everything you did and all the drugs that you may have used. When one eventually becomes a partner and have invested in the business, one soon realises how much this missed booking affects your profit and loss account, what you manage to take out of the business yourself.

But *"A Day in the life!"*

It would be nice to recall some of those busy, hectic, and enjoyable days back in East Devon at the start of my career, but I guess at that stage of my career I did not have the inclination to follow James Herriot and eventually write a book of my memoirs. Of those glorious days in the beautiful Devon countryside and those wonderful Devonian farmers, wonderful times which set the roots for my career path. I also guess that in those former years, I had a great dislike of writing, stemming from past school and university days, there was no way that I would ever be authoring a book, let alone several. So, I never made any notes, and my memory is not good enough now to recall those happy days. Certain incidents then yes, but whole days of work slipped my memory a long time ago.

And in my last few months as a vet, Covid made life so much more different from the whole of the rest of my career. I retired at the end of May 2021 but the last time that I physically went into the office at sat at my desk was March 16th, 2020. Because of social distancing and to ensure if one of the staff became infected, then they would not come in contact and spread this new disease, us vets worked from home, and it made it a far different and remote job to what had been experienced in the past. Work was quieter to as social interaction diminished to begin with, a new and not altogether enjoyable existence until after I had retired. Though it was nice to see all the office staff come outside to say goodbye on my final day.

So, from my latter years I will try and outline a typical day or two in the life of a working farm vet, something that I now sometimes miss, or is it just the farmer contact and working with them and their stock in the countryside?

I set off from home very much knowing what my day will be, at least the morning anyway. A morning starting with routine visits, regular fertility visits to farms that I went to on a regular basis to do whatever was presented for me that day. Pregnancy diagnosis, non-bullers, cows that had endometritis after calving and any sick cows, calves, whatever needed doing on that day. Plus, there may be some herd health planning as well.

My first call had been brought forward to a day earlier and I would go there straight from home to be there at eight o'clock. A herd I had been going too for some years, a pedigree Jersey herd where I had developed a good working relationship with the head herdsman and his wife who looked after the calves. It would be a sad day for me, as they had decided with so many changes in management that they had had enough of the farm and had decided to move on, ironically to my beloved Dorset to take charge of a dairy herd down there. It would be my last routine visit with the herdsman, next time I would see someone else.

Sometimes this visit would take half an hour, sometimes a lot longer depending on the number of cows that were to be presented, but it was a good handling system where we could line fifteen cows along a race with the cows at a slight diagonal so I could go from one to the next to the next in no time at all. All we did have to make sure of was that working through them so quickly, that all the information was recorded about the right cow and that she received the correct treatment if any was required.

When I arrived, David told me he had a lot of cows in today, just to tidy everything up for the next person to be taking charge. Many of the cows would be PDs to check whether they were in calf, some to confirm how far they were as there were two service dates. It was a straightforward visit, filling the race then I would scan the cows one by one as David recorded the results. Having completed the row, I would then treat any that needed it and then we would empty the race and refill it, repeating the process. The pleasant thing about this system was that there was a metal bar that fitted over the rails of the race so that if it were not full then one could move this bar to behind the last cow, keeping them compact and easy to work with.

The herd was divided into two to fit in with the housing accommodation available which meant we had two groups of cows to go through. But it was a good system and in just over an hour I had got through fifty cows, and we were done.

Having washed off and quickly discussed the results of the days mornings work it was time to say goodbye to these two people I had worked with for so long. Perhaps, abit like me, they were traditionalists and had not quite moved on with the times, and sometimes the old ways are still good, but progress goes on. It was time for them to move on for a more sedate life and me to think of how we could get this farm working to its true potential. That would be for another day.

But I had finished in plenty of time to get to my next routine visit which would start at ten o'clock prompt and one I never wanted to be late for. This was my biggest client with a massive herd split into two calving blocks. It was always a busy routine where I would be seeing anywhere between twenty and forty cows each fortnight. We attempted to keep a tight calving pattern to fit in with their block calving system, so cows needed to clean up as quickly as possible after calving, i.e., if they did have endometritis or had retained their afterbirth, we needed to have them ready for their next service as quickly as possible. Large groups of cows would be pregnancy diagnosed the previous evening then any not in calf I would treat at my routine, plus any that had been missed the previous evening. Sometimes, and there would always be a couple of sick cows or cows not producing as expected (in such a large herd there would always be one or two of these), we may finish off having to operate on a cow with a displaced abomasum, sometimes there would be the odd calf to look at, sometimes I would even end up having to do a calving.

But today, having arrived on time and set up what I needed by the cattle race, at ten with the arrival of Gwynn and Fiona, we were ready to start working through the large group of cattle waiting patiently for me in their groups at the far end of the race. I would examine the cows, tell Fiona any treatment that the cow needed to clean her up or to get her to come bulling then Fiona would jab the cow, me do anything that was necessary from behind the cow such as inserting intra-vaginal hormone devices. Both Fiona and Gwynn would record whatever treatment was undertaken, Gwynn like me liked his paper records, Fiona would in time enter any cow treatments onto a computer program and with her phone could instantly tell me of any previous treatments that any cow had received.

Over the next two hours we worked through all the cows, not always the nicest task as those that retained their afterbirth, with it decomposing inside the cow, did not give off the nicest of odours and even with two gloves on, the stench could work its way through and onto my arm. A smell I would carry with me for the rest of the day.

We were nearly done, I always liked to have a quick chat about what I thought of the cow bodily condition, was it causing any health or performance issues, even little things like the consistency of the faeces or how clean the cows were could give some indication as to the health of the cows, tying that in with how they were performing in milk production.

And lastly before I went, Fiona asked me just something to think about for the future was coming up with a suitable vaccination program for the heifers coming into the herd and the cows which would fit in with their system of two blocks of calving and that some of the heifers were reared and went to the bull away from the farm. We needed a manageable and robust system so that nothing would slip through the net, trying to protect them from a couple of diseases that we knew to be on the farm, existed on most dairy farms in this country.

A long but productive visit, I had finished there, and it was time to ring in to see if there were any other calls. There was, a lambing which was just over the hills from where I had just finished. This was on a farm high up in the Shropshire Hills, a farm with a harsh environment, open and exposed to the elements. I had only been there a couple of days earlier when I had had to lamb two ewes with a happy outcome of two sets of live twins.

Twenty minutes and I was there to find an ewe with a tangle of lambs inside her. Twins again, but I would just need to sort out whose legs belonged to who before extracting them from the ewe and into the world. With a little bit of fiddling about inside her, I was able to find a head and two legs belonging to each other and gently pull them forwards while gently pushing the other two legs that were there backwards. It was a big lamb but with gentle traction I soon had him out and rubbing his chest got him breathing. He started to shake his head, welcome to the world! He was ready to be placed by mum's head before I felt inside her again to find the other lamb. Again, a little fiddling about as this lamb's head was tucked behind but managing to straighten it and getting a lambing noose over the back of its head, again he was soon out, breathing, and ready to meet up with his mum. Everyone was happy, it is always nice to bring new life into the world and see them both trying to get to their feet and find their way to mum's udder for their first feed.

It had been a busy morning, time for a quick lunch at the office before heading off to another farm close to home to do some more fertility work on a big suckler herd which produced many fine pedigree animals but often by embryo transplants, producing strong genetic lines. Valuable heifer and bulls were produced to sell on to other producers wanting to improve the quality of their stock.

This would mean synchronising groups of cattle so that they could be primed to have these transplants at the same time and meaning in terms of management that these groups would be calving about the same time. The calves would be valuable and often delivered by caesarean. Today I would be seeing if the last couple of groups were in calf, any that were not then we would need to get them bulling again so that we could get them in calf again, possibly again synchronising their heats. Paul and I quickly worked through this group of cattle with successful results, we only had a couple that needed treating, which were not in calf, and a couple that he would not persist with, they would go fat to the market for beef.

At this time of year Paul would be busy lambing, again producing high quality pedigree lambs, a proportion who would be sold for breeding, others would be fattened to be sold for the lamb in our butchers. We would be constant visitors to the farm at lambing time and it was always worth enquiring what was happening that day, it may save a visit later on that day. All was quiet, Paul and I had a brief chat before I set off for what I thought would be my last call of the day, the other side of Telford.

Rob, a real character, an old-fashioned farmer who when I first knew him milked a few cows through an old-fashioned parlour but now had sold the dairy herd and just had a few suckler cows and calves, and his pride and joy, a few longhorn cattle.

He had called the practice requesting a visit for a calf with a bad eye. I was closest so the office asked me to go, and if sometimes abit of a rodeo there, it was always in my mind a fun farm to visit. Rob always liked a chat, and I knew that when we were done, it would be time for a cuppa and a chin wag.

The calf was amongst all the other cattle, so took some catching but I managed to collar her in the end, watching out for the one or two cows in the group who did not take too kindly to strangers. Pinning the calf against a wall, I managed to hold it and look at the eye which had a small area of ulceration on it. It would need an injection into the conjunctiva, so I left Rob holding the calf while I went back to the car to get what I needed. Again, a cautious return watching out for the not so friendly cows, I injected the calf and let it re-join her worried mum.

Rob said he also had a calf scouring so we had a quick look at that and as it was looking a bit dehydrated, I passed a stomach tube into it to get some fluids inside it, demonstrating to Rob how to do this so that he could do it the following morning if necessary if the calf was not sucking mum.

I had done all my calls; my day was finished other than Rob's promised cuppa. He would get his packet of fags out and light up, and enjoying the spring sunshine we chatted about farming old and new. A real character.

It was approaching five o'clock by now, it was not worth going back to the office, it would be long closed by the time I got back there. Home was closer and that is where I would go. Booking my work would have to be for another day.

It had been busy, but that is how I prefer it to be.

Another day, what will it bring? If yesterday had been a very structured day, knowing what I was doing from the off, the start of the day with routine visits, then today my itinerary would be decided by the telephone, I was the free vet so would do the fire brigade work throughout the day, the emergencies and the odd visit to any sick animal needing our attention.

So, it was not an early start and all being well I would start my day at the office, waiting for calls to come in. I would spend my time catching up on booking, any lab results that I needed to report to the farmer by phone, and just generally making sure I was up to date until directed by the girls in the office to a call.

That was the plan, but often it does not work out like that. While driving in, my parrot started talking, not a bird that drove around with me but my hands-free car phone. It was James, one of my farmers I did a routine visit to, and he had a cow calving. He had tried but was getting nowhere with trying to bring this calf out into the world. I was on my way in I told him and would just make the short diversion off my path to his farm and would let the office know what I was doing. I knew that this would have been in the middle of his milking so his day would now be running behind time if he had spent some time trying to calve the cow.

Despite being his regular vet, as I changed course towards his farm, I reflected on how few calvings I had done there considering the number of cows he had, over three hundred, and the length of time I had worked in the practice. But I knew he used a British Blue bull on a lot of his cows, and with this bull, calves could be quite large. If I had been lucky with the number of calvings there, I knew other vets from the practice had not been so lucky!

My arrival was greeted by James who took me to the cow after I had donned my waterproofs for the first time for the day. She was standing in a stall patiently waiting for someone to help her in her demise. James said he would get Chris (his herdsman) to come and give me a hand while he finished the milking. He explained that he had been trying for some time to calve the cow, he could feel the calf coming normally, front feet first but the head was turned back on itself so although the legs were in the birth canal, the head wasn't, and it wasn't going to come out as it was.

Chris arrived with a bucket of warm water, and we got on with the task at hand. I have found over the length of my career that as I have got older, and I do have long arms if not being the tallest person in the world, that cows have definitely got bigger. I lubed my arm so it would slip inside the cow's birth canal easily, lube being a vital component in the easing out of a calf, especially if the cow has been trying to calve for some time and has lost a lot of her foetal fluids. In this case she had but as my hand slipped inside her, yes, I could feel as James had described, two front feet coming towards me, but I could also feel that they were large.

"Is this a British Blue calf," I asked.

Chris answered, "Most probably."

I reached in further and again could feel what James had described, a shoulder and with a firm object disappearing in the other direction as the calf's neck was bent back on itself. With the loss of foetal fluids and the duration of the calving, I could feel that the walls of the cows uterus were starting to close down, to contract on the calf meaning there was even less room to work with, to try and manoeuvre the head around so it was pointing in the right direction, into the birth canal and out towards me.

Chris, I had worked with a lot in the past and was always interested to learn, to know what was going on so I continued a dialogue with him as to what I could feel. With my arm still inside the cow, I tried inching my hand around the calf's neck towards its forehead and if possible then along its nose and if I was lucky, I would be able to get my hand into its mouth. I think we had both realised by now, and even James when he was trying to calve the cow, that with the protracted length of calving time, the calf had died inside mum some time ago. If you pinch between a calf's toes when it is still inside mum, you will normally get a response, a reflex where it will try and withdraw its feet away from you. There was no response at all to this.

My efforts to slide my hand around its head were gaining some reward, I could go as far as its eyeballs, and then stretching in deeply could just about get my fingers into the angles of its mouth and then try and pull gently towards me. There was not enough room with the uterus contracting, I explained to Chris that I would give the cow an injection into her vein to see if that would relax the uterine muscles, and with that, hopefully I would be able to work the head around but it didn't always work especially if the muscles were getting tired.

I gave the injection, and we waited a few minutes for it to work if it was going to. I tried again, reaching inside again, reaching around the calf's head, and getting my fingers inside its mouth again. I tried with my other hand to push gently back on the calf's feet, pushing it back into the uterus to try and create a bit more space, room for me to try and bring the head around into the right direction.

If the injection had caused the muscles to relax a little, it had not made a vast difference and despite my efforts over the next few minutes, and much sweating, it was obvious that I was getting nowhere very quickly.

Chris looked at me, his expression was, had I a plan? Well, now I had three options. Firstly, I could persist in what I was trying to do over the past few minutes, but all the time the cow would be getting more distressed, the uterine muscles would be tiring more and starting to contract. Secondly, we could consider doing a caesarean, but it would be to get a dead calf out of the cow, and my third option was to do an embryotomy, to try and cut the calf up inside the cow and bring it out in bits. That sounds gruesome I know but is often the choice with a dead and especially rotten calf, where the risk of peritonitis would be high with a Caesar.

We decided we would try this, an embryotomy. If I could cut the head off the calf, then I hoped it would be possible to extract the calf then remove the head from the cow afterwards. This was always a gruesome task.

A trip back to the car to get what I needed, some embryotomy wire, a couple of handles (Health and Safety wouldn't like it but I found a couple of hoof knives a comfortable grip to attach the wire to, then holding on to their wooden handles) and an aluminium tube I had acquired on another farm many years ago, part of a milk pipe, which I would run the wire through so that when sawing, it would protect the sides of the birth canal from the wire.

With a loop made in one end on the wire, it was time to reach back inside the cow, taking the wire with me and trying to thread it over the top of the calf's neck, not entirely easy with the muscles contracting the walls of the uterus down onto it fast. But with a lot of effort, I did manage to push it down through the crooked neck. Then it was a matter of reaching under the neck to try and retrieve my loop and pull it gently through and back out of the cow again. It was tiring work but at last success and threading the wire through my metal tube and attaching one of my hoof knives on each end, it was now time for the challenging work. A firm stance and then grasping each handle, using those shoulder muscles backwards and forwards in a sawing motion as the wire worked its way through the neck of the calf.

I think I was getting too old for this, maybe the next one I will get the farmer to do this part and I will offer advice!

There is that wonderful feeling when the tension suddenly goes, you know you are through, and it is time to try and calve the cow again.

Putting my hand back in, there was almost a relief as one felt the calf coming towards you, further than it had been before and attaching the calving ropes to its front feet, with a little traction, we soon had what did transpire to be a big calf now out of the cow, though headless.

I reached back inside, trying to find the head which I did and turning it around and grasping it by the lower jaw, I was able to now remove that as well. Success over what had seemed an age but in fact was only forty-five minutes, a tiring start to the day, but if a little gruesome, at least we had an outcome. Antibiotics and an anti-inflammatory injection and we were finished.

Milking now finished, James reappeared with a welcome cup of coffee while I cleaned myself up.

I would phone in and see what they had waiting for me next.

It was a long drive in completely the opposite direction, in fact with a little thought I would be going back past home and towards Bridgnorth. Richard was one of our newer clients, having joined us from a neighbouring practice. He had a wonderful herd of pedigree Holsteins and was now starting to turn over the running of the herd to his son and daughter. The whole family were very pleasant and cared plenty for the health and welfare of their herd.

Today he had rung the office with a cow which had a nasty mastitis, an infection in her udder. I was on my way, heading towards the farm though the journey would take me a good forty minutes. I was greeted by the daughter, and gathering my equipment, she led me towards the cattle yards and to where the cow was. We got her in from the straw yard she was in and secured her in one of the farms examination stalls. This was a sad looking cow, breathing heavily and it was a real effort for her to walk. She certainly was a sick cow. It was explained to me that she was usually one of the first cows in the parlour for morning milking but today she had come in last, and that was only after the cowman having to get her in. She refused the food, the cattle nuts she would normally get when being milked, she was lethargic and her udder felt firm and swollen. On stripping milk from one of her teats, I found that there were clots in the milk and it looked a little watery compared with what milk usually looks like. She had mastitis and it looked a bad one so the vet, me, was summoned to treat her.

I went through my routine of examination of this poorly looking cow while she just stood there looking miserable. Temperature, nothing spectacular, but then with severe mastitis cases it can rise very rapidly then fall just as quickly dropping to subnormal as the infection turns into a toxaemia. Her rumen was not turning over, her faeces a slightly yellowy colour and on the loose side and then examining her udder, things were changing.

What had been white and watery not so long ago at milking was now clear, like serum in just the one quarter. The udder over this quarter was reddening and looked angry. This looked like a rapidly developing toxic E. coli mastitis which can often be fatal if not treated quickly and aggressively. Antibiotics into her bloodstream and here we had to be selective as in the past we had experienced antibiotic resistance to a certain drug, anti-inflammatories which would help combat the toxaemia and make the cow feel better in herself. A sort of cow paracetamol!

Then importantly in what we had found makes a far better prognosis to these cases than when I first started in practice all those years ago was the administration of copious amounts of fluids and electrolytes by stomach tube. In severe cases where the cow is down, then strong saline solutions can be given intravenously, getting some fluids into the system before giving fluids by mouth, she was not quite that bad. Difficult through the railings of the stall but I managed to pass a stomach tube down her oesophagus and into her rumen, and then with the pump attached to the stomach tube, administer twenty-five litres of fluids into her. Instructions were left to strip as much of the infected milk out of the quarter before letting her back into her straw yard so she could rest and try and recover. I was hopeful that the infection had been spotted soon enough that she was not too toxic, and that would enable a good recovery. The farmer would give more fluids in the evening and repeat the antibiotics the following two days. But I would speak to them the next day to see how we were progressing and of what course to follow.

It is surprising how a seemingly so sick cow, on the administration of anti-inflammatories, can so suddenly regain her appetite and it was encouraging to see the cow go back into her yard and start looking for silage to eat. Fingers crossed; all would be well.

A phone call the next day, and the cow was making a brilliant recovery, was eating again and the milk was starting to look like milk again. A good result.

For me, now back in the car, what would my next call be? It was lambing time and although I had always much enjoyed this time of year, there was always one farm that I dreaded going to. This was not because it was a horrible place to go, it was just because if you were in a hurry or had to visit late at night when bed was calling, it was always a hard place to get away from, the lady who owned this flock liked to talk, and talk, and talk!

I was heading back towards Shrewsbury again when the parrot rang again and directed me towards Vera's on the outskirts of town. Yes, it was a yearling ewe having difficulty in lambing. From past experience on this farm, sometimes you were called out and it was easy, all that was needed was another pair of hands and after a quick examination you would soon have two live lambs taking their first breaths in the pen, and soon on their feet looking for their first feed from an ever eager mum. All one then had to do was to escape as Vera chatted and chatted and chatted. You would manage to get back in the car eventually and open the window to say goodbye. A big mistake, she would in an instant have her head through the window and continue her conversation. I am told I have the patience of a saint but at times it was sorely tested, especially as I said, late at night or if you had another call to go to.

On other occasions, I had arrived in the lambing shed to find the patient was not much bigger than the newly born lamb in the next pen. A slight exaggeration, yes, but some of these sheep were too small to be carrying lambs and be able to lamb them normally, they would have been the late born female lambs from the previous year, but the ram was not going to say no!

This was one such occasion, and looking at the ewe, even before I had examined her and I was resigned to the fact that I would be doing a Caesar here, and that meant doing it by myself while Vera continued her conversation, leaning against the pen fence. I examined the ewe, could hardly get my hand through her birth canal and as I had suspected, the only way this lamb was coming into this world was out of the side of mum.

From here on in I knew I would be doing everything myself while my hostess, a dear old lady but probably lonely would relate any and every story about Shropshire life to me. I would have to find some bales of hay or straw to make my operating table, better than having to kneel over the sheep on the floor, less back breaking, and then I would have to find some baler twine to secure my patient to the "table". Luckily, there were straw bales close at hand, ready to provide clean bedding for the sheep and as they were still the old-fashioned type of bale, small and handleable by one person, there was also a readily available supply of twine. I made my operating table, attached two lots of twine to some rails at the back and then had to roughly move the ewe by myself on to it. Lucky she was a light ewe, otherwise I would have been struggling by myself. I secured her there with the twine, laying it across her behind her shoulders and in front of her hips, also immobilising her legs while I tied her down. She was not going to go anywhere quickly.

By now, my narrator leaning over the rails was telling me why the local livestock market, no more than a stone's throw from where we were, was not successful and why she used the market at Market Drayton instead. In years gone by, if you mentioned a town in Shropshire then there had been a livestock market there, but with changing times, alas no more!

Removing the wool from her flank, the ewe that is, I was ready to clip her up and then clean my operation site ready for the surgery that I was about to commence. I have described the operation in *"The Quiet Vet"* and so will not repeat myself, other than I was doing it with only one pair of hands, my own, there was no assistant to help me revive the lamb or anything else that I may need a hand with.

My patient was behaving herself and I got on with the task at hand, I was through into the ewe's abdomen and searching around for a leg to incise over through the uterine wall. By now we were discussing, I say we as it was a one-person conversation, local planning permission, the loss of green and brown belt land, and all those farmers that were now long gone. The changing landscape.

I produced a lamb, still alive, but needing a little help to get it going and this is where another pair of hands would have been good, I would lose my sterility in trying to get it going but it could not be helped. The lamb was alive and breathing, it was time to now sew up the wounds while listening to what the neighbours were getting planning permission for on their farm, a big poultry unit so she had heard. I nodded my acknowledgement while continuing the operation, there would not be many minutes now until I would be finished.

I had finished, and while I cleaned the ewe up and released her from her bonds I listened to the state of TB in the county, this lady knew everything! I wanted to see the lamb up and sucking, getting its colostrum from mum, ensuring it got a good start in life so held mum while showing the lamb her teats. It, it was a female, wanted to suck readily and mum did not object either. Thankfully for such a young mum, it looked like she had all her maternal instincts, all would be well.

All I had to do now was to give her some injections, clear up my equipment, remove my operating table and after washing myself off, try and escape. I just had this feeling that everything I had been listening to I had heard the last time I was here and probably the time before that, doing a caesarean on a small ewe again then. Again, my patience was a blessing.

I was washed and ready to go, all I had to do was to actually go and past experience had told me this wasn't going to be a quick process. But a saviour arrived, and if it meant more work on what was turning out to be a busy day, was I pleased to hear my phone ring with the office now requesting me to be elsewhere. I had the excuse to be able to get into the car and go, another emergency.

A dear old lady, and you must admire her for still farming with all her years, a way of life! But always a time-consuming call. I just hoped that in twelve months' time that I would not be there again doing a caesarean on the little lamb that I had just brought into the world.

I was back in the car and on my way to another sheep call, this time about fifteen miles away, a ram that had cuts his face open badly and needed stitching. This time, a family new to farming, they were actually in the building trade but fancied some of their own stock and over the past few years we had treated their pigs, now cattle and sheep. I had already been there several times earlier in the year for quite a few lambings. Today something different, but straight forward. Clean the wound up and then after giving a little local anaesthetic I was able to close the wound, technology, we now had these staple guns which were great for this type of case and made a very neat job of closing the wound. Twenty minutes and I was done and having probably driven the best part of a hundred and fifty miles already today, was ready for a short break and some lunch.

But that lunch would be brief!

A call had just come in for a calving, I would soon be on the road again to this farm near Newport, I was certainly going to be clocking up more miles in the car going here. A beef suckler herd, another farm that was newish to us as the farmer had moved up from the Southwest to start this new enterprise. I had spent a morning some weeks ago pregnancy diagnosing all his cattle on what had been a successful session, showing that the bulls had been doing a good job. Amongst his commercial suckler cows there were a few pedigrees amongst them, in the future there may be a project to enlarge the pedigree herd.

I arrived at the farm to be directed down a farm track, thankfully concreted, towards the cattle handling facilities, a series of catching pens and a race with a cattle crush at the end of it, one of the better ones where the sides can be taken off if necessary giving full access to all parts of the occupant. There waiting for me was Mick, the farm manager, and his helper along with an Angus heifer, my patient. Sticking out behind her I could see two enormous feet.

Mick told me that she had been trying to calve for a considerable time and that what I could see now, there had been no progress from this now for a long time. He had put his hand inside her to feel the calf and had tried assisting the calving, but again without success. He had called me out!

Our patient did not seem to appreciate that I was there to try and help her, and it took a considerable effort on our behalf's to eventually get her into the cattle crush and for me to try and examine her. She was not happy and in no way appreciated my presence with her. But in between her jumping about and swishing her faeces covered tail across my face, I did manage to get my hand into her and feel for myself what was holding up the calving process. It was patently obvious that this calf was big, far too big to be able to squeeze through her pelvis. The calf was coming backwards but even from its feet I could see it was large, feeling inside, the width of its hips was far too large to come out, too large even to engage in the heifer's pelvis.

We would be doing a caesarean again, this time on a cow. We were outside, down a track and the weather was not looking that special. The sun had gone in and there was a chilly wind blowing, and we were exposed to it. But that was what it was so I would just have to get on with it where we were. The lad was sent to get me some hot water and I started to prepare for the operation, clipping up my surgical site and then thoroughly cleaning it when my water arrived. This is where this type of crush is great because we could take all the metal work down on the left-hand side of the cow while she was still restrained in the head yolk. I would have to give her local anaesthetic into her flank, the site I had prepared to operate from, and one would have to admit it was no cow's favourite occupation to have needles inserted into her side. My heifer was no exception with her taking great delight in trying to kick me. I did succeed in between the swinging foot in my direction, and we were finally ready to open her up and try and remove this calf. Sadly, we were pretty sure that the calf had already died in this protracted birth.

The heifer gave up trying to fight us and eventually lay down, whether that made it any easier or not I am not sure but at least she couldn't kick me if lying.

Again I am not going to describe a blow by blow account of the operation, only to say that once I had opened the uterus and found some front legs to pull on, we then saw how big this calf was, it was enormous and thankfully we hadn't tried pulling it out through the birth canal, it could have damaged the heifer permanently.

It took the strength of all three of us to withdraw the calf from the heifer's side, having to enlarge my incision a bit to allow this to happen. Yes, it was dead but at least the heifer was not damaged. All I had to do was to sew up the uterus and then the flank layers, arduous work on the back leaning over her all that time and by now getting colder and colder. The wind had got up and it was a bitter April day with the odd shower blowing across.

I was at last finished, cleaned the heifer up as best we could and gave her what medication she needed. It was time to release her from the crush and let her return to her mates who were standing around in the field near the pen wandering what all the fuss was about. Me, I then had to clean myself up which was not the nicest task in the bitter wind. Oh, the life of a farm vet.

I left Mick with instructions on what the heifer needed over the next couple of days. She was back with her mates and did not particularly look that worried about the ordeal she had just been through. A bite of grass and all is forgotten!

For me it was now back to the office. Would there be any more call today, I was on call in the evening. All was quiet, at least for the time being, I could clean up properly, get my Caesar kits washed ready to be resterilised and restock anything I had used today to replenish supplies, plus pick up another couple of surgical kits, just in case.

I would hope for a quiet night, but it did not auger well when on my home yet another call, this time to a sick cow. Luckily, I had not got too far on my way home and was able to turn around and head off to this call. Something relatively straightforward, a cow off her food who had recently calved and was easily dealt with using that stomach pump to get some fluids and nutrients into her to restore her bodily requirements. Again, washing myself off, I set off towards home again with fingers crossed my days' work may have finished.

Well, I did get home and I did get my supper by which time it was getting dark. The phone rang again, a cow with her bed out and annoyingly only a couple of miles from where my last call had been. I was back in the car again and thankfully with the evening traffic now diminishing, it did not take me that long to get to the farm to be greeted by the upper echelons of the farm management, the farmer, his son and the head herdsman.

I was led into a barn where a cow was sprawled out on her side, newborn calf nearby, and behind the cow this grossly distended red bag, her uterus which was now turned inside out behind her. She was a massive cow and wedged against an interior wall, it was lucky we had so many hands to help because she was going to have to move for me to be able to put her in a position that I could try and rectify her predicament. Between the four of us and with much grunting and straining, we managed to push, pull, drag her away from the wall and then get her into a position that I could replace the prolapsed uterus.

First job was to prepare a site antiseptically near her tail base and then to administer an epidural anaesthetic to her which would stop her straining against me as I tried to push the uterus back inside her from where it came. Once that was concluded, there was not a lot my helpers could do other than watch, but they were a group of people I had always got on well with and so while I worked, we had an enjoyable and light-hearted conversation. For me, it was a matter of lifting all the uterus up in my arms as high as I could and letting some of the blood that was engorging its layers drain away before trying to manoeuvre it back inside the cow, trying to invert it while doing so back into its natural state. Slowly but surely, I was winning until I reached that satisfying moment when you feel it all suddenly disappear inside, I had won. One does have to check that the uterine horns are fully inverted, and I have described in *"The Quiet Vet"* the use of a Reisling bottle to facilitate this. All was good so again after giving the cow the necessary medication, I was done and just needed to clean myself off before heading home again. It is a messy procedure, and you often look as if you have been at some sort of massacre when you are done, covered in blood. I have often wondered what would happen if stopped by the police on the way home and they saw you in this state, try as you might you never seem to get yourself spotless, especially washing in the dark. But I had done my best and it was time to go. It had been enjoyable; the farmers were great company and we had got a good outcome.

I think I would soon be ready for bed, but it would not be long after I got home that the phone would go once again. How many prolapsed uteri do I see in a year, certainly not that many? One a month, probably not even that many but now I had two in the same evening, and I would be making that journey back towards Shrewsbury once again.

I had been to this farm before but some time ago and it had been in daylight. I knew it had two entrances, one each off two main roads but could not exactly remember where. The farmer had given me rough instructions how to find the place but the directions he had given me were from the opposite way that I had been before. Where I was supposed to turn left, I turned right and was some way down this track before I realised that I was not going to come out at the farm where I thought I would. I had to turn around and retrace my path before joining the main road and trying to find the right track in the dark, not really sure where it was. And when I did find the right track, it went on forever and again I was starting to doubt myself until I saw some farm building lights in the distance.

I was there at last. This prolapse, a heifer who had just calved and carrying on straining until her inverted uterus followed the calf out, turned out to be far simpler. She was still standing, waiting patiently in the cattle crush for me, and again after administering an epidural, once I started to try and replace the uterus, it was only too keen to return to its normal position inside the heifer. This time it did not take many minutes and I was soon washing myself off yet again. A good job done, and I would try to get home again.

I did and was glad of my bed. The rest of the evening, night was undisturbed. Had I driven many miles today, over three hundred and I made a mental note that first thing in the morning I must fill the car up again. A busy but fulfilling day, and in the next couple of days I would have two more prolapses to deal with as well as a couple more cow caesareans.

Even after that many years as a farm vet, you can never be sure what the next day will bring. But then, perhaps that is part of what makes the job so interesting and fulfilling. Two spring days remarkably busy, very different.

My old days in Devon were always busy but I think that is the way of these small family farms where each cow is so important to them. We have taught farmers to do a lot themselves so a lot of that work that I did then has gone. Now on some summer days, you would spend just waiting for the phone to ring if you did not have routine work already arranged. Some days would be incredibly quiet, catching up on reading, research, drafting articles for our monthly newsletter.

Even over forty plus years, every day was always different and there was always the unexpected that may happen, a strange case, something you had never seen and I guess with that you are never too old to learn.

THE BEAUTIFUL
GAME:

BUILDING UP RELATIONSHIPS to me has always been an important part of my job, in fact in any job one needs to build a level of trust with both your fellow workers and your clients. As I have said before, times have changed in my time as a vet when starting out as opposed to the new graduate these days. We, all those forty plus years ago, left University with a degree and were expected to function as a vet from day one in our first job. Now, you will work under some sort of guidance or internship to protect you from some of the stresses now faced by an ever-demanding public. You may have learnt some of the skills in your latter years at university, especially if you had been seeing practice somewhere that helped you develop those skills needed while you were still a student, but the first time you had to carry out an operation or consultation by yourself, it was still very daunting.

But communication became increasingly important to establish that trust, that client/vet relationship and to make sure that what you had said was fully understood so that there could be no come back on you as to what was or may have been said.

The arrival on my first farm when I was qualified, stepping out of my car to be greeted by a farmer sceptical about this green vet who had just arrived to examine one of his financial assets. I was a farmer's son and had much experience of life on a farm, but I was shy, lacked a bit of confidence and so still was more than nervous about case number one! What was my best bet? To try and get the fact that I was a dairy farmer's son into the conversation as soon as possible by making a comment about his farm and how that compared with dad's. It broke the ice, gave us something in common to talk about, but I still had to back that chat up with competence on the farm with whatever I had been called out to see. As I have mentioned many times in my early experiences in Devon, that would involve lame cows and there would always be disappointment, whatever the cause, if the vet did not find some pus in the affected foot. Puncture wounds were common from stones or nails lying about, common things occur commonly as we were always taught at university by Jim Pinsent, so pus was what was expected!

Sport always is a good medium for stirring conversation. I was a hockey player and so after a while, did join Exeter Hockey Club which ran a single team, and then joining another Exeter team which did have a small farming contingent playing for it. I did get to know some of my farmers better through this, playing with them or their sons had broken down some barriers.

While I was in Devon, I met some of my now lifelong friends, but their sport was rugby, playing for Taunton further up the M5 motorway. We did get together to watch the as it was then, Five Nations, the ladies often watching with us while enjoying a bottle of wine, a white German "Crown of Crowns". How one's tastes change over the years, wouldn't touch it now even if it still exists. We even went to Twickenham a couple of times to get in those days, our annual trashing by the Welsh. What a joy in 1980 to win the Grand Slam, and there was that famous match we watched, the girls may have idolised Nick Jeavons and Peter Winterbottom, but us men, Erica Roe, cheered up our afternoon!

And in those days, we did get to see the All Blacks playing Southwest Counties in Exeter and go to the old Arms Park to see them again in a third place play off in the Rugby World Cup. Something to talk to my farmers about!

I had played a little rugby for the Vet School in my last year at university and I was persuaded to turn out for my pub against another pub side which turned out to be Tiverton Second XV in what was a friendly, and from what I can remember was in aid of some charity. I played in my favourite position of scrum half, and all was going well, with several farmers, or sons of, in our side. Again, good client relations, but friendly, one of my vet colleagues who was recovering from a bad ankle had to be carted off to the local hospital, shortly followed by one of my best mates for life, Anthony, who had one collar bone in two bits sticking in opposite directions. Again, the girls were carting another of our team off to the hospital. And finally, another of my mates accidentally kicked me in the head in a maul. As I staggered to my feet slightly concussed, I heard him say to the rest of the team, "Come on boys, we must give Rod more protection."

I finished the match; we were well in the lead at half time but with our fast-depleting numbers we held on to win by one score.

But it did keep me in touch with the farming community present, scoring a try in the game plus a few brownie points in their eyes as their vet. I was even asked to play for Tiverton afterwards, but the thought of only playing two weeks in three and recovering from the knocks and bruises afterwards, I stuck to hockey.

So, sport after Devon, I was involved still, again mainly through the local hockey side and again there was the odd member of the farming community who played but it was not until I moved to Shropshire that sport really played some part in building those client relationships that are so important. But there was a local interest especially when Exeter City had a good cup run in the very early eighties. An interest in football was suddenly sparked amongst the farming community, keen now to discuss the merits of their local team, I had never heard a mention of them before. And who did I live next door to, Martin, the Exeter right back. Next door to him, Ray and Nina, a lovely couple who we spent many hours with, him a striker for City. Just up the road, Pete, Martin's brother and the midfield dynamo. next door to Ray, Vince, the Torquay goalkeeper. We were surrounded by the local football talent and much conversation would start from that.

Let me hang my colours on the wall now, I am a Man Utd fan, have been since watching them in the '63 final against Leicester

City. The days of Charlton, Law, Best, there to name a few. My son followed my interest in the side, then my daughter too and through a friend we did get to see some games at Old Trafford. The kids enjoyed in and of course at that time the title was ours most years, we went, we won, and the kids were happy. I at last managed to get season tickets, two were expensive enough so could only take either Richard or Lydia to each game. Mid-week, then I had a couple of farmers locally who were keen to go, or if I were on call, they would take both tickets.

For one of them at one game, I had tickets about ten rows back near the goal line, and when the ball was cleared into touch, one of those funny incidents but may be not if you were the one affected, a ball hurtling at a great rate of knots into the crowd, the person in front of my farmer friend moving out of the way at the last moment for the ball to hit my ticket holder straight in the face. And another time, they always had a half time draw and the prize was £2K for the first prize, £1K for the second. I had a feeling it was my turn, the first number was drawn, not me. The second number, yes, it was mine but then it was announced the prize was a flight in a helicopter over the ground. Was I disappointed, so much so that I sent my twelve-year-old daughter down to collect our prize, being presented by some rock star. She made her way down and walked along the side line in front of the south stand to the halfway line. The rock star greeted her, full of himself, said to her, "You know who I am don't you?"

"No," she replied in front of seventy-five thousand plus spectators, "I have no idea!"

Light laughter went right around Old Trafford.

When I moved to my final job outside Shrewsbury, I was of course a very experienced vet by then, but still felt a little apprehensive starting out in a new job with new clients. I suppose I was in the initial stages of my developing depression then. A monthly newsletter went out and any new member of staff would be asked to write a short bit about themselves in it, a bit of background, family, and hobbies. Whatever you wanted to say about yourself, so here was the opportunity to say I was a farmer's son, where I had worked before and my interests in playing golf and watching football and rugby. I stated that I was a Manchester United Season Ticket holder.

It was surprising just outside Shrewsbury how many Man Utd fans there were as farmers, also a similar number of their arch-rivals, Liverpool. On arriving on a farm of one of my new clients, I would be greeted with "you're the United fan aren't you."

A slightly hesitant "Yes" reply not knowing if the farmer was for or against, we were winning the title most years at this time. And the likes of Neil, Les, Bill, and many others were like minded as me, keen supporters. Two especially, Pete and his son Chris who had also had season tickets but due to the time pressures of dairy farming and milking, found they no longer had time to go so had given them up.

So, while examining the farmer's cow we could discuss the merits of the latest performance from *Match of the Day*, or a live game on TV and it soon broke down the barriers between farmer and the new, old vet. Even more interest when the farmers found that I had season tickets and could not always go so Bill and his grandson would always be willing recipients to go in my place. And their friends knew that they had gone and had used my tickets so that provoked further conversation as to how pleased they were that another lifelong fan was now able to go in there latter years.

My football interest was creating many conversations, interest in me and my support, "the beautiful game". I do often wonder where it got that name from, "the beautiful game", a game kicking a round object around a pitch hoping to score a goal or two. Tribal instincts amongst fans which was often associated with crowd violence and certainly at times, far from gentlemanly conduct on the field of play. I would often go and watch my son play as a teenager and would be acutely embarrassed at fellow parents shouting abuse at opposition parents and players, "kick the b......d" and other such friendly comments. The rivalry in the stands at Old Trafford, some light-hearted banter, some singing and some of the chanting was just downright hatred. For heaven's sake, it was only a game.

But those days of supporting and winning were enjoyable, especially having time there with my children, especially my daughter when my son had gone to university. We could discuss the likes of Beckham, Scholes and many others but especially Cristiano Ronaldo who in my mind (even if he is letting himself down now) is the best footballer I have ever seen.

But I suppose as depression started to affect me, at times I would sit in the stand and after twenty minutes or so, would think what am I doing here? Certainly, as far as going to live matches, my interest was waning, Bill was happier to take my tickets more often but still there would be that focus of conversation about football when visiting farms.

United peaked and fell, then it was the time for those Liverpool fans to come more out of the woodwork, they were at last enjoying a much needed revival and the likes of Graham at Forton would be only too pleased to greet me on my arrival on farm with their latest win against us, or our latest loss against anybody. It was all very light-hearted but though rival fans; we established a working relationship through our football interests. There would be the odd Chelsea fan I would meet on the way, even a few Wolves fans merged as they regained a degree of success, won the Championship, and returned to the Premier League. I never could stand the colour of their shirts! In time it was nice even to find a couple of Shrewsbury Town fans, local farmers taking themselves off to support their local team on a Saturday afternoon, the game played at that traditional time of the week, unlike my United support which was never at that time.

I gave up my United Season Tickets, I was finding football a frustrating game to watch, especially as I have just said, when I was diagnosed with depression. Was it the game, the amount of time it took to get there and back and because my daughter was less able to join me as she worked and had a family, I am not sure. I would have to admit it is rare for me to watch a game now, too much passing sideways and backwards, too much obscene money in the game. United were not doing so well but the interest from afar was still there, was happy to talk to farmers about them, the international team, whoever. I wasn't a glory fan, I had supported them through relegation, through good times and bad but I guess as time went on and especially with Wasps (a team I had followed for many years and had travelled down to High Wycombe to see them play many times) moving to Coventry, my interests were turning more towards Rugby Union.

I had been keen on watching Internationals for many years, always trying to make sure I was not working on now Six Nations weekends. In Wenlock I had worked with Ben Kane, a vet who gave up his career to become a successful writer of historical novels, who was just as keen, if not a keener rugby fan though he was Irish and this produced more than a little rivalry in the office especially for one fixture a year.

But again, many farmers, or more specifically their sons also play rugby and as I worked in Shrewsbury, I found a few that played for the local town, more who went down the road and played for Bishops Castle. I had found another group of farmers where there was a common interest and this would provide a topic of conversation while we were castrating a group of eighty calves, or just something to talk about when we had finished our business and over a cup of coffee or while cleaning up it broke down the barriers and I was able to build up a good client/vet relationship with them.

In the office I was surrounded by a group of vets who also enjoyed rugby, some still turning out for the local team, others like me who just now enjoyed watching. An Irish contingent again, a Scot, a Welshman and several English supporters meant a lot of friendly rivalry amongst us all. Even one or two of the ladies in the office, Vicky especially going to many Internationals, were keen supporters too. Come World Cups there would be a sweepstake raising money for such charities as *Mind*, where everyone would join in, drawing a team. I was never going to win with Tonga, I cannot remember who it was who wanted their team and not the one they had drawn. Rosa, one of Spanish vets who knew nothing about rugby nor that Spain played the game, had the team he wanted and asked her to swop. She did, ending up with South Africa and so ended up winning our little office draw.

In time I would get Season Tickets to see Wasps in Coventry, my wife, Jane, had decided she liked seeing burley men running around in shorts, and at the time, Wasps were certainly an exciting team to watch. Unlike at Old Trafford, we did seem to meet the same people each game in our row of seats, like minded ticket holders, and could build up a relationship with them, and they were always interested in who were in our seats if we could not go. My farmers did use my tickets on several occasions to take their sons to see a top rugby game live, and how they enjoyed it would be reported back to me next time I went to their farm.

So, rugby also played an important place in breaking down those barriers, giving me and client something to chat about informally during or after work. Sport in general, there is generally a common interest in there somewhere, football and rugby especially.

One or two farmers, the ones who were Shrewsbury Town supporters in fact, who I never realised were that interested in sport, and I would later find out how they were big cricket fans. They were going to take me to Edgbaston but sadly we never got around to it before David passed away through cancer, but like me in my youth turning out for the local town team, joined by several farmers, they too in earlier days enjoyed their Saturday and Sunday afternoons playing with the red ball. Interestingly though, the biggest cricket fan I found in my years in practice was one of the pharmaceutical reps, Kath, an avid fan who would watch as much cricket as she could.

Sport, especially football and rugby, made me many friends in my time as a vet and played more than big part in developing those lasting relationships I had with so many clients.

The beautiful game!

COTTAGE FARM:

LIKE DRURY LANE that I described in *The Quiet Vet*, there were always some farms I always looked forward to going to, even if some of these farms were infrequently. Cottage Farm was always one of those.

David, I have mentioned in the previous chapter through his interest in the local football team and for his love of cricket. But both these facts I found out only in the latter years that I knew him and gave us more topics of conversation as we enjoyed that well-earned cuppa after we had finished whatever work I had been doing for him.

Cottage Farm reminded me a bit of my dad's farm in his early days. He farmed there with his wife, Gwyneth, always a happy and welcoming farmers wife, always interested in my family and my wellbeing. They had a disabled son who spent most of his time in a wheelchair, with impaired speech, but again always pleased to see you and interested in David's cows. He had developed an interest in old Massey Fergusson tractors, and he spent many hours doing them up with help from friends and was always so pleased when you showed an interest in them and asked him what he was doing.

But although some of the farm had moved with the times, some had not. David inherited and had worked with his father in producing a top-quality Jersey herd of just under a hundred cows. Both had made their name in Jersey pedigree circles and David would boast how he had beaten the Queen in various breed classes throughout the country. The farm had progressed to a cubicle building so each cow could lie in her own individual space, but the parlour was still from the dark ages. It was an old fashioned shippen, a line of stalls split between two buildings where these small jerseys would come in, tied in their stalls while they were milked and then released back into their feeding yard while the next batch would come into the parlour. Thirty at a time, milking was a slow process especially as there were no standings, the cows were at ground level and so were you when you were milking them. A back breaking job when you were young and certainly no joke when you became older.

But this hundred cow herd was like having a hundred pet cows. Yes, they produced milk commercially, high in butter fat content and cream, but they were also just so friendly. They had been bucket-reared as calves by Gwyneth and so had no fear of humans, in fact were only too pleased to see you. If you entered their pen then they would mob towards you thinking it was feeding time again and whatever you were trying to do would be hindered by numerous tongues licking around you, searching for any food you may have on you that they fancied. You would end up soaked, covered in calf saliva! It would often be the case that if you were doing anything like Tb testing the cows, then rather than having to run them all through the parlour, taking care to inject them all the same side, you would just go into the yards, David would walk up to the cow, put his arm gently around her neck, I would do whatever I had to do before he released his hold and would move onto the next one. Such friendly cows, with each having their own name, but whether Health and Safety would allow that now, I am sure the Risk Assessment would probably say no!

In the latter years of him having cattle, we did run them all through a cattle crush. But they would all still be so quiet and calm to the point where they became a bit of a hinderance to you as they wanted to come and inspect you while you were doing something else to their mates. A lovely, lovely traditional herd producing milk in a very traditional way, all well looked after and cared for by more than able stockmen the likes of which are very rare these days. All you did have to be wary of were the Jersey bulls, I had long ago been taught never to trust one, should you trust any bull? Certainly not a Jersey however friendly it may seem. Few would reach old age as they had turned nasty by then. David, they knew, but even he respected their temperament, would never let you go into a pen first even if the bull was tied up.

I would pull up into the yard, always parking my car beside the straw rick in front of four loose boxes, step out of the car and start changing into boots and waterproofs. It would never be long before David would appear if he was not in his office opposite where I parked the car.

He would always greet me, "How are you, Rod?" followed soon after by his reply as if I had asked the same question, "Alright thank you".

A bucket of hot water would soon appear in one of those old-fashioned galvanised metal buckets plus soap and water and would be positioned just inside the entrance to the parlour ready for when I needed it. Then, whether we were working in the parlour, through the crush, or just catching cattle where they stood, I would help him move the cattle to where we wanted them.

Those bulging eyes, those long drooping eye lashes looking at you, inquisitive to know what you had come for today, their orange/yellow coats and darker faces, beautiful cows and so well suited to the farming system that David ran.

David was always characterised by the flat cap he wore; did I ever see him without it? I do not think so. Proper trousers, never jeans, and in his check shirt, he was a traditional farmer, even still possessing one of those hand and bow seed drills that I do not think I had seen since dad had one in the fifties. A vegetable patch just outside the yard would grow wonderful vegetables for the family to eat in the house, this really was a traditional, old fashioned English farm set in the middle of a small Shropshire village, where the locals would come and chat over the farm gate. There was always time to be friendly and sociable.

Most of my visits there would be routine over the thirty years I attended. Every time I moved practice, David followed me to my new one. Generally, I would be going to pregnancy diagnose his cows and heifers, to disbud his calves and for the annual TB test. I saw the occasional downer cow there, Milk fever being the commonest cause, a breed failing but they all did get up in the end. In my early years when visiting, we did see several cows with ketosis, a metabolic crisis soon after calving with the odd displaced abomasum, and opening these cows up, operating on them, would be amazed how much fatty tissue they contained within, always of a yellow colour. If you didn't know the breed you would have thought they were jaundiced.

But I think in all those years of visiting Cottage Farm, I never did one calving there. Jerseys are an easy calving breed and my experiences on the farm backed that up. Because he used his own bull, invariably all calves were jerseys, small calves weighing twenty, twenty-five kilos and no problem just to be popped out.

As I have said, it was always a pleasure to go there, probably very few of the other vets in all those years ever visited as he would always ask for me. A true bond between farmer and his vet. We did have the odd disease outbreak, scouring calves, a touch of pneumonia now and again but in general the herd stayed extremely healthy. I think the only thing that I never did solve, stop, something common on old fashioned farms was the use of a bucket of warm water and a cloth to wipe the cow's udder and teats clean before the milking machine was applied. It started off hot, and even if it did have a bit of hypochlorite in it as a disinfectant, this same cloth would be taken and used on every cow that was milked. The water got cooler, the disinfectant became less affective, the cloth got dirtier, it was a potential disaster. It was a recognised method of spreading bugs from one cow to the next, a potent way of spreading contagious mastitis pathogens such as Staph, aureus. But as much as I tried and as much as David had a few cows that became chronically affected, I could never persuade him that that damned cloth was the cause of the infection spreading from cow to cow. In the farming community, sometimes tradition overrules all, his dad had used a cloth and he was going to continue to do so. In general, now, most dairy farms use paper towels from a dispenser to clean the teats, disposing of it after each cow, hence no spread of bugs from one cow to the next.

But like his cap, he was never going to change.

Sadly, for the family farm, his son Peter was never going to be able to take it over from him. There reached a time where as he got older, and all that bending down to do the milking was becoming too much for an ageing back, he reached a time where he decided the cows would have to be sold, he couldn't go on any longer as a dairy farmer and wanted to spend more time with his wife and looking after Peter. The decision was hard, but it was made, and he arranged to have a herd dispersal sale in Beeston market. Tuberculosis was rife in the county, and to have a sale he needed to have the herd pre-movement tested before they could be sold, within sixty days of the sale.

The test was arranged just before the planned sale date and if it was a sad day anyway as it marked the end of the herd, it became even sadder when we found that there were Tb reactors present. All those years where he and his father had been clear, and now when it really mattered, he had the disease in his cattle. The affected ones would have to go for compulsory slaughter, the rest would need three clear tests before a sale could take place, which would mean three tests minimum, sixty days apart so if no more failures, the earliest the cows could be sold would be in six months' time. Autumn was approaching and not expecting to have any cows on the farm, David had not done what he had done every year until then, he had not made any silage or hay, conserved forage to feed the stock over the winter.

Disaster, this really was a disaster now, and it could not have happened to a nicer, kinder person who so really cared for his stock. Thankfully, local farmers rallied around to distress calls and eventually David managed to get enough forage to see him through the approaching winter when his cattle would be housed and would still be milking. The farming community had got together to help one of its real gentlemen.

For a while he seemed like a broken man. His retirement plans had taken a bit of a hit, but he was a real Trojan, if down to begin with, he had a herd of cows still that needed looking after, milking and feeding every day. Life would have to go on until he was free of this cursed disease in his herd when he could think about selling again and giving him and his family the easier life they deserved after all those years. He would have to get through the winter, continue milking as before and he still had his friend up the road who would help with that, and feed as best he could. Perhaps the quality of feed he now had was not quite of the quality he and his cows were used to but that was what he had, and he was eternally grateful to those that had helped him out.

My work would continue as before, the occasional sick cow but more commonly doing fertility work to check that the cows were in calf, and the now dreaded intra-dermal skin test that would occur to test for bovine Tuberculosis.

Sixty days passed and I was back on the farm for the first Short Interval test. It was a worrying day for the family, would they go clear this time or would there be more reactors, requiring compulsory slaughter. Going back three days after injecting the cows with Avian and Bovine Tuberculin, (it is a comparative test seeing if there is any difference in reaction to them, measuring skin thickness then again on the return visit at the injection sites) it was time to read the test. David was a great stockman, he knew his cows and I knew he would have looked at all their necks for lumps, reactions, and probably had some idea of what the result of the herd test would be, but it was up to me to read it properly and decide whether he, the herd had passed.

It was a more subdued affair than it had been in the past, a great deal rested on this and subsequent tests. We went through the herd one by one, looking for these skin reactions. Thankfully, this time as we neared the end of the test, cows done and with just a few calves to do, it looked promising that the herd would be free, at least for the time being. There was a huge sigh of relief when we finished the last animal, one of the breeding bulls where extra care would be needed because of his temperament, but the herd had passed. There were the odd skin reactions to measure, but none where the bovine site had reacted to the Tuberculin more than the Avian.

Stage one had been passed but David would still require two more clear tests before he could consider selling the herd again, two more tests sixty days apart and the worry would persist until after then as long as each test was clear, longer if they were not. It would be an anxious wait. We arranged the days to repeat the test two months hence and would keep our fingers crossed for then.

I took my friend Sally to help me the next time, while I did the test she would do all the clerical work, recording the skin measurements of each cow as I took them, ticking each cow and calf off the list to ensure every animal had been accounted for, tested, so that when we submitted the test to the powers that be, we could tick the box that it was a clear test.

Again, the return three days later to read the test, and even if all these beautiful cows were getting a bit apprehensive about that stranger coming and sticking needles in them on day one, by the third day they were only too pleased to see me again, coming up to sniff and lick me while they waited their turn to be read. They were always such lovely cows to work with and thankfully again after a nervous wait to conclude the test, I could inform David that all was clear again. Sixty days would see me back to do hopefully the third and final test, by which time it would be spring and time to turn the cows out to grass which would at least alleviate some of the feeding problems, stretching out what available forage he had managed to get to last him through the winter.

Accompanied by Sally again, not only was she good and helpful at doing the clerical work but also had that human touch to help all through that worrying time of testing, calming nerves, and it never hurt to have a bit of glamour on farm! The whole farm was anxious, on day one when I injected, but even more so when we returned on the third day to read, interpret the test. That job of examining the neck of each animal, looking for lumps, skin reactions to the Tuberculin and measuring them if necessary. Each time I took out my callipers to measure a skin reaction there would be worried looks on the faces of David and Jim, his helper. On this occasion, every time I measured then I would reassure them that there were skin lumps but that this cow had passed the test and on we would go to the next one until there were none left.

It was a clear test again, that was the three and David was now free to arrange to sell the herd again, but it would have to be done within sixty days of this test or else we would have to test the cows again, this time as a pre-movement test, a requirement for cattle to try and limit the spread of disease throughout the country.

A preliminary date had been arranged with the auctioneers, it just needed confirming after the test to say all could go ahead. A sigh of relief all round, but celebration I am not sure. Yes, David could now contemplate selling the herd in just a few weeks now, but there also had to be a sadness of the finality, confirmation of the sale would mean the end of David and his father's life's work in the building up and the breeding involved in such an outstanding herd of Jerseys, and the reputation that it had made. But we had got there, we had got through all the necessary tests, and we had got through the winter. The cows had been fed well, had milked and were healthy. That to David as a good stockman was as important as anything.

I would see him and Gwyneth from time to time before the sale date was due, just making sure that all going to the sale were healthy and fit. It would seem that my duties and vetting adventures at Cottage Farm would be now coming to an end.

But as the sale neared, it just seemed to be the right thing to do to go and support David at his sale and so I asked work if it was possible for me to do that, client relations and all that, otherwise I would take it as a day's holiday. They were extremely happy to oblige, these were people who had been clients of mine now for many years, and when I had changed practice, they had followed me. They had been so loyal to me and now it was my turn to return some of that loyalty by just being there for them at this nostalgic time.

Sally had become a friend there as well helping with testing and being a shoulder to cry on when things had not gone well. I asked her if she wanted to come to the sale at Beeston Market as well, she was only too pleased to say yes. So having done a couple of calls in the first part of the morning, I picked up Sally and we took ourselves up to the sale. An hour or so drive on a dull, overcast spring day and we were there to observe the hub bub of a cattle sale by auction, not something I had seen since I was a kid with my father.

The sale was under way by the time we arrived, the cows going into the ring one by one, Lot 10, Lot 11 and so on. We sat in the stands watching, observing as each Lot came up. What was a good price or not we hadn't a clue, sales can be strange things and it all depended who was there, which farmers from renowned herds or those trying to improve their own, might even a representative from the Queen's own herd be there looking to purchase one of these fine pedigree cows? There would be a couple of things which may discourage bidders, especially the fact that it was well known that David's herd had gone down with Tuberculosis as the sale had already been postponed, and the shortage of forage had been well publicised.

So, as I said, were these decent prices the cows were making (and this would be David and Gwyneth's pension fund)? Personally, I thought the cows would fetch more money, there did seem a couple of bidders who were buying a lot of the cows but at a price favouring them, not David.

We went to find a cup of coffee, and to find David if we could. I saw him in the distance wandering around and went to have a chat with him. It was an emotional day for him, and it showed. I said did he want a cup of coffee and a walk, and having found refreshment I think he was quite glad that Sally and I took him away from the sale, away from the dispersal of his life's work and just chatted the other side of the carpark about anything he wanted to, keeping his mind off the sale. If he was a little tearful when we first bumped into him, he was smiling and talkative after a while and glad to see some friendly faces.

It was the least I could do for a good client who also had become a good friend. We couldn't stay to the complete end of the sale but at least thought that we had gone, that we had given David some support, and a break from it all, if only for a few minutes. I hope it made his day more bearable for him.

A life's work gone at the drop of a hammer. He would know a lot of the breeders that had bought some of his cattle which were soon departing Beeston in large livestock lorries to their new homes. One hoped that they would be so well looked after, cared for as they had been by David and Gwyneth, and in return would perform for their new owners as they had at Cottage Farm. They had been a well contented herd and always had been a pleasure to work with, I would miss them.

David could now spend some time adjusting to a new life, no early morning milking, nor evening spent in the parlour, that back breaking parlour as he was getting no younger. Time to pursue some of those other interests he had, the ones that at that moment, I did not know he had.

Would I see him for a while, which was an interesting question, we had few other clients in that direction, but I would go out of my way to call in and catch up when the opportunity arose. I did get a phone call from him a few days after the sale thanking me (and Sally) for sparing the time and making the effort to attend the sale. He said that he really appreciated us taking him away from it all for a while as he had found it hard seeing his cows for the last time before they departed to pastures new. For now, he was going to take himself and Gwyneth, Peter too, on a well-earned break for a few days to recharge his batteries, and to take his mind off not getting up to deal with the cows and calves. I thought that was a wise decision, and on his return would be interested to know what his plans were for the future.

It would be a few weeks before I heard from him again, me getting a message at work to see if I could give him a ring. When I spoke to him, I guess he confirmed what I had already suspected. He had been in farming all his life and he wasn't about to change now. He had decided that he had two choices, he could rent his ground out for grass keep but would still have time on his hands to kill. Or he could use his land and buildings, offering his services as a heifer rearer for another farmer, having their youngstock from weaning until they were due to calve when they would return to their mother farm. This would give him an income, an interest and keep him occupied though not fully. He thought this an ideal solution going forward, and in asking my advice I could only agree with him. I guess I thought, like so many other farmers, it was in his blood, and he wouldn't be happy if he wasn't doing something with livestock. And Gwyneth would be extremely willing to help look after the calves as well, to go hand in hand with tending her Shetland ponies.

It was decided, he had a plan going forward and just wanted a little advice on control of a couple of diseases that may crop up, originating from the main herd elsewhere. He had been approached by another Jersey breeder and so would be happy to continue working with the breed he had known and loved all his life, and to which the farm had been adapted to. The cow's cubicles could be used for in-calf heifers, the rest of the lean-to open fronted sheds could be used for the younger calves, giving them shelter, warmth, and comfort.

The workload necessary to look after these calves and heifers wouldn't be over taxing, feeding them twice a day, a few minutes every day scraping the muck out from those sheds that needed it, and just generally keeping an eye on all the stock. An ideal world for David, still some farming life for him but also giving enough time to now pursue his other interests, those that he had struggled to do over his farming life.

My role in his farming life would not change that much, the important goal for him was to get the calves to grow quickly and be in calf ready to fit into the calving pattern of the home farm where all the stock originated from. Therefore, unless anything was ill, and that was an unusual event, then I would be checking to see if the heifers were in calf, scanning a group when there were fifteen or twenty to do, treating any that had not been seen bulling, and of course the routine six monthly Tuberculosis tests as required by law.

Everything was running smoothly, David was happy, the owners of the stock were happy and for me, it was always a pleasant visit, to enjoy their company, listening to them all talking, discussing the pedigrees of their stock, and listening to David talk about his hobbies. It was about this time that I discovered his interest in sport, especially football (Shrewsbury Town) and cricket where I found out that he was a member of Warwickshire County Cricket Club. Many interesting chats would ensue after we had finished our livestock work and while washing up and enjoying a cup of tea with him. If there was one blot on the landscape having at last reached the time to enjoy time together away from farming, it was becoming obvious that Gwyneth was showing the early signs of dementia. She would always seem to be so happy, would come and chat with a big smile on her face, but showed alarming unawareness of the dangers that handling cattle could throw up. Sometimes she would position herself in the middle of the yard while big animals were running either side of her and it got worrying for us to try and move the cattle around but be patient with her as she put herself in dangerous positions.

It gave David a lot to cope with, both with her dementia but also Peter's handicap, he could not look after himself. David would be grateful for those friends that came round to help Peter with his hobby of doing up his Massey Fergusson tractors, of which he was getting quite a collection.

One of the countryside's really nice people but having to endure so much and always with a smile on his face. Always so polite and so kind, a real gentleman.

So, what he did not need was more problems with the stock he was looking after. It was midsummer and it was time for his six-month Tb test again, which worked roughly in line with that of the parent herd. Sometimes this test would be done by their vets, then I would do those at David's, at other times it would be the youngstock done first by me. This time it was us going first, a hundred or so stock to test ranging from young calves to heavily pregnant heifers.

David had got all the stock in from their respective fields so all I had to do was to turn up and do the test, group by group and as ever, the first day when I was injecting them with Tuberculin, all went smoothly. I returned three days later to do the reading of the test, and to begin with all was going well.

But David had one group of heifers which at the time were grazing a field the other side of the road from the farm. These were the pregnant heifers, and he was feeding this group of eighteen supplementary feed, cattle nuts, feeding them in low metal troughs just above ground level. It was their turn to be read and even from a distance I could see that there were going to be problems, I could see large skin lumps at my injection sites even without having to get the cattle into the cattle crush. One by one they came through and one by one I read them and found in several of them that there was significant reaction. He had Tb on the farm again in his cattle. Of the eighteen, eleven had significant reactions, in fact they were Tb failures, reactors, and with that as a Notifiable disease they would have to be culled. Furthermore, restrictions would be put on the farm preventing movement on and off the farm until there had been three clear tests again.

The biggest impact here other than losing valuable herd replacements was that as the farm was now "shut down" for movements and the parent farm was still classed as clear. What would happen when the heavily in calf heifers that had passed the test had calved? They needed to be at the parent farm to be milked, but would be stuck where they were, unless there was some way that an isolation unit could be set up so that there could be no risk of them spreading disease to other cows if they were moved. This was unlikely to be allowed, nor would young calves be able to move the other way, onto this farm in case they would be exposed and catch Tb.

The problem was solved when the parent farm also had a

reactor at their next test shortly afterwards, not good news for them but at least it solved a potential welfare problem as the movement of stock between the two farms would now be allowed under special licence.

It had been just one group of animals at Cottage Farm that the problem had arose in, and sadly the most important group as they were all pregnant. I do not want to go into the rights and wrongs of badger culls here, but badgers had been seen in the field and had been seen feeding out of the troughs. In hindsight David realised that he should have had troughs above badger height so that they would not have been able to access the heifer's food in them. There was a clear implication that badgers were involved in this disease cycle, but now the surviving seven heifers from the group would be housed in isolation from the rest of the stock. Only time would tell as to if others in the group had been infected, I would be testing again in two months and again in two months until we had got our three clear tests again.

Those tests followed at the right time and if there were no problems in the rest of the stock, this group continued to be a source of worry. Seven left, after the next test there were three, the next test and just one remained and despite their continuing to be problems at the parent farm, Cottage Farm would go clear after that last test of two reactors. Those three subsequent tests, all clear as it turned out but a huge worry for all involved until we did finally get that final clear test.

A group of eighteen and only one did not succumb, only one was able to calve and go into milk production. This had been a great emotional trauma to all concerned. Happily, in the end, the parent farm went clear as well and some sort of normality returned to life, my visits to see David would become the pleasurable visits they had been before and I would find out more of his other interests, his cricket, and his football.

But it would be nice to say there was a happy end to all this. David was one of the nicest farmers I had met, a real old-fashioned gentleman but fortune did not want to favour him. Gwyneth's health, her dementia would continue to deteriorate to the extent that she would have to go into a care home. David had the stock and Peter to look after, impacting on his time to be able to pursue his other interests. Then he became ill, and it soon became obvious that this was not going to be a passing condition. He was admitted to hospital for tests and sadly was diagnosed with cancer. His deterioration was rapid, coming home but soon being readmitted. Others helped back home with the stock and with looking after Pete.

David soon died without ever really having the time that he would have liked to enjoy with his family, or the free time to follow his interests as much as he would have liked.

I went to his funeral and smiled as on his coffin was a framed photograph of his Jerseys but also placed prominently, his flat cap that he had worn for all those years that I had known him. He would take that cap to his afterlife. There was a wonderful tribute given to him before his final journey.

A farmer I shall never forget.

BACK to BASICS:

COTTAGE FARM, DAVID's farm with his beloved Jerseys was a throwback to the more traditional methods of farming going on when I was brought up and being practised on many of those small family farms that I worked on when I started my career in Devon. That traditional method of dairy farming was that of producing milk off grass, a low input, low output system of milk production practiced over hundreds of years previously. It was a relatively low-cost system with labour being provided by the family and maybe one or two others. Tied cottages may have been provided and your hired labour tended to be very loyal. You tried to calve your cows in spring, early summer when grass was growing well and the cows grazed pastures lush with the green stuff, so as they reached peak production, then there was plenty of nutrition growing outside to sustain that production. Any excess, and there would be, could be made into silage or hay to provide nutrition during those chilly winter months when the cows would be kept inside. Break crops such as kale was grown for winter feeding as an alternative, which when finished could be ploughed and then reseeded to produce fresh grass pastures. Again, a relatively cheap fodder which allowed for some sort of crop rotation which is good for the land.

There would also be the old meadows, lined with hedgerows full of songbirds, the odd large tree breaking up the landscape, and in those meadows an abundance of flowers, buttercups, plantains, dandelions, even orchids I can remember which also gave life for an environment for insects, butterflies, and bees. That was what it was like in those smallholdings in Devon and on many of the surrounding dairy farms in Berkshire when I was growing up.

Happy days in glorious countryside, cows happily grazing with not a care in the world. They ate, they milked and when the time was right, they produced another calf, and the cycle would all start again. Indeed, happy days and perhaps that ideological scene is how the general public would like to think their pinta (or should I say litre or half litre) was produced, full of cream, especially if it came from the likes of David's Jerseys with their high butterfat content. Those old-fashioned milk bottles delivered by a milkman, leaving bottle on your doorstep, and for those bottles of full cream milk, there would be Bluetits only too happy to peck through the silver foil top to have their share of the cream provided. Those were the days, certainly the days of when I grew up though my milk came straight out of our first churns, and then our own bulk milk tank, ready chilled to give longer life.

Dad's system was slightly different in that although we tried to feed the cows on as much grass as possible, and the farm grew grass better than anything else, we suffered from a series of droughts, the soil just wouldn't retain what little rain we got in the shadows of the Berkshire Downs. His was a more of an intensive dairy farm, he could be considered somewhat of a pioneer in intensive farming. To make farming pay he had to produce as much milk as he could from as many cows as he could stock on the farm. This meant feeding a lot of bought in feed, high in energy and protein.

This was the early seventies in the last century, farming was changing with more and more intensive farming methods, greater costs in production which would be rewarded with greater yields. One just hoped that the rewards for production was a decent price for the products produced from the farm. A Milk Marketing Board negotiated for the dairy producer to get a fair price, but under the Thatcher years, the Board was declared a monopoly, was disbanded and quotas introduced as to how much milk you could produce at a premium price. Various milk purchasers were set up who you could have a contract with for them to purchase their milk. This of course set up competition along with the growing power of supermarket chains so as milk was often sold as a loss leader in store, the price to the farmer often suffered and milk production became harder as margins became tighter. We got to the state where certainly for the small family farm, they could not afford to compete against the big producers who could to some extent dilute their costs. We started to see the decline of the dairy industry as more and more milk producers sold up their herds and found alternative sources of income, many switching to beef production.

As vets, did this affect us much. Probably not in terms of practice income as we adapted our work away from the fire brigade work of before, and more into routine fertility and herd management, fixed work on a regular basis, working hand in hand with the dairy producer to increase production to sustain their place in the market. Changes in management style, changes in breed to the more productive Holsteins, often imported from across the water. These larger cows, with greater production potential led to substantial changes in production methods, their feeding requirements were different. There was no way they could eat enough grass to sustain the milk production potential they had so there was a trend to growing maize to feed them on, a high energy feed, high energy density so their dry matter intake could match their predicted production levels. And of course, this changed the landscape of the country, especially in those parts of the country where the climate was suitable to grow maize. Fields got bigger, machinery to plant and harvest these crops got bigger, some of the beauty of the countryside was sacrificed to support the needs of more modern farming. Hedgerows were lost, trees (if they had not been ravaged by the likes of Dutch Elm disease) were felled to make the use of these machines easier.

High level use of inorganic fertilisers became increasingly common to try and maximise crop production, both in grass growth and for cereal production including maize.

Farming had changed but somewhere along the way there was a group of farmers who wished for the "old" ways, producing food from the land without adding artificial ways of production.

Fertilisers would be organic which usually meant they came out of the backsides of cows (mixed with the straw that they were bedded on, manure) which would be spread on the land at certain times of the year generally in the early spring, allowing natural production whilst improving the quality of the soil formation, in our biology days at school, humus. A soil where the likes of worms and insects became increasingly important, a return to nature!

The ORGANIC MOVEMENT was beginning with certainly a part of the population, the consumer, welcoming this reversion to old methods and being happy to pay a premium for food that was produced in the way that they wished.

Here in Shropshire, throughout my time here, I have attended a few of the same farms in every practice I have worked for. Allan, Angela and James's farm was one I have worked with throughout that time, also working alongside their herdsman Chris who over the years has become a good friend. In 1998 they made the decision that they would go to organic milk production and would have to undergo a two-year conversion period. This would mean producing milk under organic principles but still getting the milk price for conventional milk production.

What changes would they have to make? To begin with to maximise milk production in an organic way, they would have to produce milk essentially from grass and that would mean the cows would need to be producing when grass growth was at its peak which would mean that they would need to be calving in late winter so that at a period some thirty to forty days into lactation when they should be reaching their peak yield, that needed to coincide with the flush of spring grass as the weather got warmer in March and April. As their yields dropped in the autumn, grass growth and as a nutrient its quality would be falling so the two would be in harmony, meaning the cows could be dried off in winter ready for calving early the next year and the cycle would restart.

A different type of cow would be needed, getting away from the Holstein breeding of the past and going back to the more old-fashioned traditional British breeds, Jerseys, British Friesians along with a few continental cattle, Montbeliards from France, a dual purpose breed but one which would produce milk from grass.

The use of artificial fertilisers would have to stop, reverting to good old manure. The use of weedkillers, insecticides which could affect the ecosystem at ground level, affecting the likes of beetles which would help breakdown manure, would have to stop. More permanent pastures were encouraged, rich in clover which would function as a natural source of nitrogen capture, helping to increase the fertility of the soil.

Importantly from a veterinary point of view, the use of antibiotics and other drugs was discouraged meaning that management techniques would have to change, animal husbandry would have to be better, more care to stockmanship and that good old TLC. We would be allowed to use drugs with the proviso that if a cow received more than three treatments in any given lactation then it would be classed as non-organic. Three strikes and you are out! This had implications for cows with chronic mastitis, repeat cases which in conventional systems would require multiple treatments and even then, a cure may not be reached.

The use of anthelmintics, wormers, in youngstock was also a no-no. Parasite worm burdens would have to be controlled by pasture management so that youngstock would have a minimum contact with these parasitic worms by pasture rotation, meaning they had a little contact to build up some natural immunity but not huge numbers which could cause health issues, scouring and weight loss and even permanent gut damage. Similar control would be needed against "Husk", lungworm which could seriously damage a calf's health permanently, even kill it. There was, still is, a vaccine against it which could be used, but in the face of infection then the only treatment would be to use an anthelmintic and to do that the farmer would have to get a derogation through his vet, me, to worm the cattle and kill the infection.

The three strikes rule meant that if a cow had reached this, then her milk could not go in to the bulk tank with the rest of the cows, she would have to be managed differently and that essentially meant that it was difficult for her to stay in the herd, she would have to be culled.

So, there were a lot of changes to consider and manage and some of those involved me as a vet. How would we manage mastitis? How would we manage fertility, getting the cows back in calf and to get a tighter calving pattern to get them calving at the right time of year? And of course, how would we manage disease or more importantly how could we prevent disease? All these required a lot of thought and so a lot of my work became advisory in terms of achieving these results. I suppose from my point of view it was good to get back to good old animal husbandry and care like I was brought up with on dad's farm, and the one thing this did need was enough staff who were compliant with what was wanted to be achieved.

Conversion was starting towards organic production and without too many glitches was achieved after that two-year conversion period, though after going through this system we realised that we would have to tweak the system a bit. I was now working closely with my first organic producer but during the rest of my career I would get to work with increasingly, people who wanted to work to organic standards and produce a sustainable product which they hoped would become more and more popular with the consumer, you!

To that end, standards had to be thought out, exacted and then monitored and this task was undertaken by a body set up in 1994 called OMSCO, Organic Milk Suppliers Co-operative Ltd. This co-operative was set up by likeminded farmers, one hundred percent owned by them and run by them for their producers which were one hundred percent organic. Their wish, their conditions for a contract being to produce a product where production methods are herbicide and pesticide free, free of Genetically Modified products and are antibiotic free. Their aim, to give the consumer a choice in how their food is produced on a variety of farms throughout the country where every farm is different in its own way as they work in harmony with nature and with local communities. A return to traditional farming systems producing milk and other dairy products in the most sustainable way possible. They would state that organic farming, as well as being traditional, answers many of the challenges of today around food production, animal welfare and the environment. Their success would be to grow the supply and demand for organic dairy products, whilst having cows well looked after to the highest care standards and while protecting the natural environment.

Interestingly having written about Drury Lane in *"The Quiet Vet"*, was this not the same philosophy that Jill and her staff are trying to achieve but in a conventional milk production system. The differences, a slight difference in the breeding policy of the type of cow each farm wants to produce, a difference in calving pattern and a bit more lenient approach to their feeding systems and use of fertiliser so producing a bit more milk per cow but still based on a largely grass based system of production.

But over my final few years in practice, I would come across more and more farmers converting to organic production with this emphasis on the environment. Some of those herds would be quite large, two fifty to three hundred cow herds producing their own dairy replacements all on an organic system. My interaction with some of these herds would grow as my career approached its finally, but it was nice from my point of view to see a return to traditional forms of milk production while seeing the environment thrive as well. That, I must add, isn't to say that the many other farmers did not have a care for the environment they lived in, in fact there were many who cared passionately about their surroundings, their local fauna and flora, involving themselves for example in curlew conservation, and some returning to the old forms of hedge laying which gave a good environment for insect and bird life to try and thrive. The interaction between farming and nature was fascinating to observe and now I have retired is something I take more and more notice of as I have more time on my hands to do so.

But I have digressed away from my organic farm in the making. We were there, we had achieved conversion with the now benefit of a better milk price while achieving what seemed a more relaxed atmosphere on farm. There were changes that needed to be made to the management of the herd, now numbering some hundred and twenty cows, the biggest being going from an autumn calving herd to a spring calving herd. But we were on the way, except....

Seeing this better milk price, despite the cost of going organic, using organic derived feed stuffs while converting but getting the conventional milk price, a lot of other dairy farmers saw this as a good opportunity too. Getting a better milk price was the incentive to become organic when conventional milk prices were not rewarding. The result, the organic milk price collapsed. What should they do? What had seemed a sound economic decision which would also benefit the environment now did not look so clever.

Not all the land had by now been turned over to pasture, the decision was made that what was not already pastureland would be used to grow organically produced potatoes. If it rained, the soil was good enough to produce heavy crops of something that was always sought after. Diversification with cow numbers being cut back until the milk price would hopefully improve, times became hard financially, but the joint project did just about see them through these difficult times.

But there was still a will to continue the project and so some of the changes already mentioned slowly took place. Changing the calving pattern to all the year-round calving, then to spring calving herd, changing the breed type to smaller but more grass efficient cows. The Holsteins were going and there was a return to more of a Friesian type.

Dairy consultants were employed to try and increase yield on this system of milk production, but they seemed more interested in pushing feed intake, costly bought in feeds, than anything else but it was not producing the expected increase in yields. A combination of an all singing, all dancing feeding system was not working on this farm.

Imported potatoes from Israel were putting pressure on that

side of the business with buyers wanting these British potatoes harvested later and later. It was becoming impractical to continue growing them, so the decision was made to push the milk side again. Half the farm would be used for grazing and half for silage making. The changes in cow type continued with the introduction of Jerseys into the herd, bought in but bringing in with them the complication of Tuberculosis in the herd which would take some time to get rid of, although this was achieved after a long while. Further cattle, a group of heifers were bought from Ireland, the herd was now expanding rapidly with at last some reward in the milk price.

But there was one other big issue and that was the time it was taking to milk this expanding herd. Milking was taking over four and a half hours at each end of the day, far too long with cows standing in the collecting yard waiting to be milked when they should be grazing or resting. Equally that time interval put a strain on the milkers, nine hours a day in the parlour plus everything else that needed to be done in the day's routine, feeding, cleaning out, an endless list.

The parlour had become outdated, had been designed for large cows and these were getting smaller and certainly was not big enough to push the number of cows through that were now on the farm. Ten cows could be milked on one side, then ten on the other, alternating through the milking period until all was completed. With these smaller cows, especially the heifers, it was not uncommon for them to walk in then turn around in the parlour, amusing to watch but not so for the milker who wanting to be presented with the cow's udder would instead be staring face to face with the cow. The only way to overcome that was to have eleven cows in each side, but you could only milk ten of them. The parlour was enlarged slightly so a couple more could be milked each side, but you still needed that extra cow in to stop this turning. Milking, a lengthy business, a stress for the milkers, a stress for the cows.

So, a major decision was made to replace the parlour. The

family had strong connections with New Zealand and the dairy industry there so there was some knowledge of the types of parlours used over there on their grass-based units. A design was found that would suit this farm, bought over there, and imported to this country where it was eventually constructed by a Kiwi team working on a tight schedule to a get a few finished in the brief time they were here. A new site, a new parlour with vastly improved handling systems which would streamline milking, and also my visits. The aim, to reduce standing times while milking for the cows which would increase grazing and lying times for the cows. Automatic gates which would keep the cows tight so they would want to get in and out of the parlour quickly so they could then wander back down to the pasture they were grazing. That long milking period was now down to two and a quarter, two and a half hours maximum. Everyone was happy, milkers and the cows.

The milk price was good, we had now got a tight calving pattern at the time we wanted them to calve, we were achieving what we had set out to do from the start. It had taken time, but we had got there, and the expense of the new parlour was justified by the reduced pressure on all concerned.

The farm was now achieving a lot of success in what it had set out to do, produce milk on a low input, low output system. We had achieved contented cows who would wander down the field with one interest, to eat grass and from that, to produce milk. We had made further tweaks to the breeding, using further crosses, using Norwegian Red and more Jersey bloodlines, and in time will then back cross to New Zealand Jerseys and Friesians.

From my point of view as the herd vet, well, I would have to admit that my requirements on the farm had diminished, partly through what I believe was a very solid health program, but probably the greatest change was that the stresses on the cows was far less, and with that they were far more healthy. Milking routine along with this reduction in stress had reduced mastitis rates to the benefit of milk production and the time spent dealing with infections in the parlour. With a now non-antibiotic milk contract prevention was far better than cure so we tried to reduce stocking density to accompany the better parlour routines. Care and technique became important, continuing to reduce the stress on both cow and man.

Tb, as on any farm was a constant problem and as well as that, milk buyers had become more concerned about a disease caused by another Mycobacterium, that which causes Johne's Disease, a slow wasting disease of cattle but which may or may not have a link to Crone's Disease in humans. It was a disease that could be monitored regularly at times of milk recording and so we were able to produce an eradication program for this particular farm, albeit going as far as you can to say it does not exist on the farm. Such is the complexity of the disease, one can never say, "it is not on the farm".

A vet's year on a farm like this would start in February as all being well, all the cows would be dry through the winter and the parlour would not be used. February would be the time that calving started and as we had worked hard to obtain a tight calving pattern, once calving had started, it would come thick and fast. Through our bull selection I may be called to assist the odd calving, but it was only the odd one with cows and heifers calving easily, to begin with producing dairy replacement calves and then beef crosses. With the herd upto two fifty plus cows and another sixty heifers to calve we could see over a hundred and fifty calvings in our first three-week cycle. This would coincide with early grass growth so that on calving, the cows could be let out to graze. Grass growth and cover is carefully monitored, measured regularly so as not to over graze paddocks, especially if as so happens in spring we can get a brief spell of inclement weather.

Hopefully by mid-April all but a few stragglers will have calved, I may have seen the odd cow which has had calving difficulties and may have injured herself, the odd downer cow and as can happen at this time of year on a grass based system, one or two cases of Grass Staggers, Magnesium deficiency though we try to counteract this by adding Magnesium into the cows water supply. But with grass growth now so rapid, there is always the chance of getting a case or two.

There may be the odd calf or two to treat with pneumonia but in this system with the housing available and being able to maintain a low stocking density, cases are few and far between.

As we move into early summer that is when my work really begins, we have to get all these cows back in calf again, as well as next year's dairy replacement heifers. Heat observation, spotting when they are in oestrus becomes important and my role is seeing those that have not been observed and treating them as necessary to get them bulling so they can be served at the start of the breeding season. Again, we are looking to get as many cows served in as short a period as possible to maintain that tight calving pattern although after a couple of years, we did refine the system slightly, taking the calving period back slightly to early March to ensure the grass was growing. After a couple of dry years, silage at become in short supply by the end of the winter, but ensuring there was grass when they calved, that food supply necessity was alleviated. I would probably have two, maybe three sessions doing this fertility work, but we found that as we got the cows calving in better condition, then the fertility of the herd improved as well and I could treat as few as twenty or twenty-five cows, less than ten percent of the herd. That was a positive result.

Summer would pass and the only real issues that could occur is bloat, the rumen filling up with gas from rapidly fermenting forage, especially the rich clover pastures that existed on the farm. Episodes of this have been described elsewhere but having to feed straw to cows and keep them moving happened more than once, usually late at night as well as having to trocharise the severely affected cows to release the gas to save their lives. The episodes of drenching them with cooking oil and having to stay on the farm, important and helping to reduce fatalities. We tried to overcome this problem by pre-mowing the grazing pastures which makes the clover/grass mix less potent.

Having used Artificial insemination for the first bunch of

bulling cows, bulls would then run with the cows and the heifers to tidy up any late calving cows and those that may have repeated bulling. After nine weeks one would hope that everything had been served and so in early September, I would have the task of pregnancy diagnosing the whole herd with my ultrasound scanner, and believe me, putting your arm inside nearly three hundred animals in a little under three hours is tiring work. It became the norm to stop for a coffee break about halfway through to give my poor arm a chance to get some life back into it, much needed. We hoped we would get an over ninety percent success rate of cows in calf, and we generally achieved this so it gave us the opportunity to sell the less productive cows, or those that had chronic lameness or chronic mastitis, plus any that were calving too late to fit into the desired calving pattern. The heifers I would do the next day, again achieving exceptionally good results, these should be the animals that are improving the genetic potential of the herd.

We have encountered the odd problems with Vitamin deficiencies on some of the calf paddocks away from the main farm and I was interested when researching this to find that it was related to Vitamin B12 and Cobalt deficiencies, fascinating how all these nutrients interact to cause problems.

With that, with the cows in calf again my year would virtually be done. I would inspect the herd in early winter to advise on their condition, we did not want them too fat at calving, or too thin and it gave us enough time to adjust cow condition before e the herd would be dried off and the cycle would all start again.

I would monitor through the year Johne's results, somatic cell counts as an indication of mastitis, udder infections and would do an annual review of the overall herd health of the farm, which may involve some of the protocols we practised on the farm. We would work as a team to improve or sustain herd health and it was something that I found extremely rewarding over my last few years in practice.

The farm did start selling milk "at the farm gate" which meant some cows would have to be kept in milk through the winter to be able to keep the milk dispenser stocked, and this also meant that this milk would be pasteurised on farm to meet food sale standards. This is proving to be a successful avenue to follow, the public buying and refilling their own bottles from the milk dispensing machine.

So, the step into organic production has been interesting to me and has provided the opportunity to go back to good old stock management systems where reducing the stress on cows, sacrificing some milk yield to achieve this, has shown a great benefit to cow and herdsmen alike.

The benefits to nature may not have been as great as had been hoped for, but certainly with the rebuilding of hedgerows, more wildlife has been seen. With permanent pastures, more hares have been seen and with that, more birds of prey, more buzzards. The use of pre-mowing to reduce the risk of bloat may have impacted on ground laying birds, I was sad to hear that the species that inhabited dad's pastures, the Plover, Peewit or by whatever name you know it by, the herdsman had not even heard of, but they are not going to lay if a mower continually appears.

It has become a sustainable form of milk production with many rewards. It has given me the chance to join in at grass-based milk production meetings and discuss some of the problems and rewards that these farmers encounter, and one or two nice barbeques to enjoy while there.

And from here, what will change? I do have a small advisory role even in retirement and am interested to hear about the possible use of electronic collars which will help heat observation, streamline a system that is already working well, that will filter out cows automatically by opening and closing handling gates as a cow leaves the parlour after milking so that the cow can await the AI man. And of course, the use of sexed semen will mean that the farm can be more selective on those cows that they want to bred heifer replacements from.

Perhaps a more natural system of milk production but like everything, science is playing a bigger and bigger part on all farms.

It has been fun working on this and other organic farms. I will never forget doing a Tb test there through the old parlour which was quite time consuming doing the cows as they came out of the parlour. A neighbour's daughter, an attractive young lady came to help on this hot summers day and was quite a distraction standing in the yard in her wellies, hotpants and tight t-shirt. The joys of working in the countryside!

I would have to add after writing about this type of dairy farming that there is a role for this and for the more intensive high output farms producing a lot of milk from Holstein cows but whose requirements in terms of feeds are so different. Those high yields produced off maize silage, high energy density diets sustain an appreciable proportion of our daily milk requirements both in the liquid market and that which goes for manufacturing, for cheese, butter, and yoghurts. There is a place for all types of milk production to suit the type of farm it is being produced from. The veterinary input will vary from one type to another.

And the impact on the countryside, conservation and the rural landscape will be just as important to any type of farmer, the custodians of the countryside.

THE OTHER END:

IT WOULD BE a standing joke throughout my career, and I suspect so many other farm vets, that when meeting up with friends and them asking what I had been doing lately, they would always rejoice at the thought that I had spent my day, days, with my arm up a cow's backside. The withdrawn handshake greeting with them saying "I know where that hand has been", even if although a very right-handed person it was my left I used for my cattle work, they still found it highly amusing. I wonder how many times that joke was used over all my years. But they thought it funny, and of course the image of Herriot on tv doing likewise only added to the thought that that was how I spent my day. The difference I noticed was that the cows he saw seemed to be very clean, often seeing him examine them in his shirt, sleeves rolled up, and when finished just putting his jacket back on and walking away. No such luck for me, how many times did I not get covered in cow shit, very few!

But it is true, the average farm vet does spend most of his time standing behind a cow, or a sheep whether it be carrying out routine fertility work, doing rectal examinations to feel if any noticeable abnormality inside, or in bringing new life into the world whether that be a calving, lambing or farrowing. That part was always the really rewarding part of the job as long as a live offspring was the outcome.

Standing in stalls, in cattle crushes or in races then very often the only part of a cow you saw was the rear end, and with that what you would think would be the dangerous end where to an unsuspecting vet either of two feet could suddenly lash out at you, giving a painful kick to some part of your body. Surprisingly, I think

I could count on the fingers of one hand how often that happened throughout my career, usually a blow to a leg though once I did get both feet together in my chest. The farmer seemed unconcerned as I picked myself off from the floor, just expecting me to carry on from where I had just flown from.

But usually hidden from view, these farm animals do have other ends, heads and faces, and if we can't see what expression they have on those faces as we invade their other end, we do from time to time have to deal with that end.

In pigs, one would always be aware of their teeth, sharp in those cute little piglets, strong and dangerous when fully grown. A pig bite would produce a nasty wound, usually in the leg and a new pair of wellies would certainly be needed from the damage it caused. These teeth could crunch up anything and a board to separate you from them was a necessity. Some mouthing would just be playful or inquisitive, some would be nasty, and you could not take the risk of finding out which was which. Big old boars could have large canines which could protrude from the side of their mouths and could cause considerable damage if catching you or other animals with them. In times gone by I have seen some horrendous wounds inflicted on horses by pigs.

In sheep, their teeth give a good indication of age and can contribute to ill-thrift if in poor condition or are aged with the animal not able to eat properly or get good nutritious value from their diet by being unable to ruminate properly. Otherwise looking at the head of a sheep would usually be to find wounds, treat eyes, treat aural haematomas or as part of a general examination checking colour of membranes, pupillary dilation and as an aid to diagnosis of disease.

Any part of the body can suffer from similar conditions, abscesses, swellings, cuts to name but a few, and the head would be no exception. For us examining them, the main difference would be that being at the eye end, they could see you and whatever you were trying to do, and so were more intent on avoiding your attentions. A cow's head is a solid bit of equipment and being hit by her swinging head is more than a little uncomfortable, and if the cow's head hits yours, I can assure you that you know about it.

It therefore makes restraint of that end of the animal even more important, not just restraining the cow, but also the head as far as possible to minimise any excessive movement. If there was one thing we were taught early in our days as a veterinary student, it was how to put a halter on properly (even how to make one) but it was surprising how many students one had with you, and farmers who would continually put it on the wrong way, making restraint far from ideal. One would show them the correct way to put a halter on, the important bit being the fixed part that goes over the nose meaning the rest can slide to the size of the head allowing proper restraint. I had a couple of sturdy halters that lasted me throughout my career, always making sure when they had been employed on farm that before I left, they were put safely away back in the boot of my car. Farmers would be very keen to get their hands on them for their own use, it became a crusade to keep my own and they are both now put away for posterity.

But that restraint became ever more important especially when having to examine eyes. Both sheep and cattle are very prone to ocular disease, from trauma to infections of the surface of the cornea. Lambs could often be born with an entropion where the eyelids are turned inwards, rubbing on and causing irritation and ulceration. Cattle can be affected similarly with a condition called New Forest Eye, an infection carried by flies which if untreated could cause severe damage to the eye, even loss of it. There are eye ointments which are applied to its surface and do work if caught early enough, but in more serious cases and often there would be more than one case then we would have to inject antibiotic sub-conjunctively into the affected side. Sticking a needle into that site, so close to the eyeball could be a nerve-racking experience without proper restraint with the potential hazard of damaging the eye permanently. Thankfully, that never happened to me!

Eyes always presented a challenge right through my career, including at university. I remember in our second-year degree exams in Anatomy being set a question about the Canals of Schlemm in the eye. It was a compulsory question, twenty percent of the marks on that paper, and would have been great if I had ever heard of them. Did we have any lectures mentioning them, not that I or other members of my year could remember. I made up an answer with what knowledge of the eye that I had, did it get me any marks, I have my doubts. In the not-too-distant past it did get me a pointless answer in the afore named TV program, but that was of little value to me and probably the only time in my whole career that I needed that snippet of information.

So, I qualified and through the years would have dealings with eyes other than the common New Forest disease mentioned above. Ulceration and conjunctivitis are both common problems in small animal medicine, especially in those brachycephalic breeds where the eyeballs are so prominent. The odd permanent damage where removal would be the only option was not infrequent and with a fully anaesthetised dog or cat was quite a straightforward operation. It was surprising how quickly they got accustomed to only having sight on one side.

An operation where you stitched the third eyelid, the nictitans, over the surface of the eyeball became a recognised piece of surgery for helping to cure deep-seated ulcers and it did seem to work, removing the suture after a length of time to usually find a complete cure.

In farm work, this was more challenging as I have said earlier, performing these operations on a conscious patient. Suturing the third eyelid was done under local anaesthetic and was a little easier when we could get hold of anaesthetic drops to put in the eye to help numb it. Was it as successful as in small animal work, probably not because generally the lesion may have been too far advanced when first seen, and post-op care on a cow is a bit more difficult, you can't put an Elizabethan collar on a cow to stop her rubbing and it is harder to keep the area clean.

Hereford cows especially are prone to carcinomas of their third eyelid and removal of as much of the tumour as possible would be carried out, dissecting it out with a pair of scissors. One did have to warn though that it would almost certainly recur and sooner or later the cow would have to be destroyed because of it becoming too invasive.

Enucleation, removal of a diseased eye was far more of a challenge in a cow that in an anaesthetised dog or cat, and probably one of the bloodiest ops we would perform. As I have said, restraint would be in a crush with a halter, and probably a pair of bulldogs in the cow's nose as a distraction from what you were doing to her. The local anaesthetic was the challenge, using a long-bent needle to go around the eyeball in the eye socket to reach the optic nerve where it arises out of the skull. Not something pleasant to perform, nor that pleasant for the cow but having succeeded in numbing the area then one would stitch the eyelids together before then dissecting around them and deep into the socket, separating connective tissue and the eye muscles before reaching the nerve and blood vessels. One would do ones best to tie them off, but this was a bloody op, they did bleed well and before suturing the skin edges together one would have to pack the now empty eye socket with absorbable material which filled the dead space, absorbed some of the blood and acted as a medium for it to clot in. Before the advent of these materials, we would use an ordinary bandage with an end protruding from one end of the wound, just drawing a little out very day until all was removed, and the wound would then heal over. Infection was common then. It certainly was not the prettiest site seeing a one-eyed cow with blood staining down from the medial canthus of where her eye used to be. But again, once it all was healed, cows quickly adapted to being one eyed.

The only real hazard that eyes would present is if there were cataracts developing. Cattle, sheep, are herd animals and will follow each other. Where cataracts developed and their sight was greatly diminished, again they would manage if following the herd. The risks occurred if they became separated and would panic if they could not see, that was where danger could occur to us, the people attending them and would become unsafe to keep these animals. One certainly could not have a blind cow going through a milking parlour.

Ears were less challenging, the odd torn ear from catching it on something or where an ear tag, the official means of identifying them, became ripped out causing much bleeding. Otherwise, the occasional abscess, aural haematoma but nothing that was too much of concern or that required much in the way of treatment.

Heads did sometimes get trapped in things, a cow putting her head through the bars of a gate, panicking, and lifting it off its hinges and then panicking more as she ran around with the gate on her head. Some of the gates especially in cattle crushes are quite heavy and trying to remove them from a cow's head can be difficult, firstly because she is panicking, then you have to restrain her and she already has your main form of restraint stuck on her head and then trying to avoid being clobbered by the gate as she swings her head about. Were sedatives any help, not always as one had to worry that if the cow went down with the gate around her neck, she may strangulate herself before you could save her.

And that takes us to her mouth!

The hole at the front end where they eat from, drink from and a useful orifice for administering medicines through. Pigs I have already described and we would have as little to do as possible to their mouths because they can give a nasty bite, are not that easy to examine and to be honest other than trimming tusks, there do not generally tend to be too many problems in that part of a pig's anatomy.

But the mouth of a sheep and especially a cow we would spend much time working with. But before I consider the trials and tribulations I have had especially with cattle, I think it best just to give a quick description of the mouth of a ruminant, and by definition therefore, a herbivore. Firstly, unlike us, dogs, cats, even pigs, they have no canine teeth, they are grazers and chewers. They also have no incisors in their upper jaw, instead having a dental pad, a hard piece of tissue along the front of the mouth that lower incisors meet with allowing ruminants to pull, rip herbage into their mouths which they will then chew with their rows of molar teeth. These will grind the herbage down and in the process on rumination, when boluses of herbage are regurgitated back into the mouth, the mastication process continues while being mixed with copious amounts of saliva which aid the digestion of the food and also acts as a buffer in the pH of the stomach contents. These teeth are continually growing and being worn down with the vast amounts of work they have to do in a ruminant's life. There is also a long tongue which can grab grass, swoop up coarser meals, and if a cow starts licking you, you soon realise how rough this is. It is quite bulbous at the back of the oral cavity, the significance of which will become apparent a bit later in my tale.

What is important here though as I have already mentioned is that to examine inside the mouth, or to give medicines orally, it does require a considerable amount of restraint, and more than a little strength. Modern crushes do have gadgets which come under the cow's chin, offering a great deal of restraint and do take some of the effort out of any procedures you may be trying to do, but they are a help, not the complete answer. It certainly stops the swinging backwards and forwards, and sideways, that can be a test of your strength against the cows, even more so a bull. But for those of us that lack a few inches in height like me, and especially as the modern Holstein cow gets taller and taller, difficulties still do arise in looking into a cow's mouth or trying to administer drugs down that orifice.

Some of the ailments of their mouth and throat can be assessed from an external examination, is there swelling, excessive drooling meaning there is some irritation, or they cannot swallow properly. There are some wonderfully named conditions affecting the tongue and jaws caused by bacteria, *"Wooden Tongue"* and *"Lumpy Jaw"*, infections caused by bacterial invasion down from penetrations to the tongue or spreading down through tooth roots causing a proliferation of bony tissue in the jaw. Sometimes difficult conditions to treat, especially in jaw infections where antibiotics have difficulty reaching to the focus of infection, sometimes having to go back to the old-fashioned remedies of injecting the cow with iodine intravenously which can be hazardous itself. Old conditions which still do occur from time to time but not as often as when I started out all those years ago.

And of course, being the place where food enters the body, there is every chance of cows and sheep picking up foreign bodies while they eat. Silage harvesters may not be choosy what they pick up and of course in mown grass there will be thistles, other plants with spikey extremities, bits of branches, twigs especially after hedge cutting has taken place. All these which can either penetrate sensitive tissues or especially in the case of twigs, get stuck, embedding themselves in the sides or roof of the mouth or getting trapped across the roof of the mouth between the two sets of molars. Painful for the cow, stopping her eating properly as well and not the easiest things to remove as they do become well and truly wedged.

But what has probably caused most "fun" has been the feeding of root crops to ruminants, especially to cattle. Stubble turnips are a common winter feed for sheep, them grazing them where they grow in the field but with their incisors managing to bite bits small enough to swallow, they do not cause a lot of trouble. Cattle are fed beet, but again these roots are large enough that they need to be bitten to eat so rarely causing any problems. The potato is another story. Every year there will be many of this crop which do not grade for the supermarkets through being slightly damaged, too small, or just peculiar shapes. These become a waste product and will go for animal, cattle, feed. Some of these will go into mixer wagons, being chopped up and incorporated in a complete ration, others will just be added to the feed direct into the feed trough. They are a rich source of starch, and the cow will search through her diet to sort these "sweets" out and it is an amusing sight to watch a cow munching on a huge piece of beet, savouring the taste as she masticates in small enough to swallow. But potatoes, that is where the problems often occur, some will be large but not large enough that they cannot be swallowed and that is where the problem lies. From the back of the throat down into the oesophagus and then into the rumen, except, as the oesophagus enters the thorax between the first set of ribs, that space narrows considerably. A large potato will travel so far and then if too large to go through this space, it causes a blockage.

It was a cold February day when Anthony rang into the office saying he had a cow with choke. That invariably in a cow meant that there was something stuck not in her airway but in her oesophagus. I had already that winter been to this farm a couple of times, and I was not the only vet in the practice to have done so, to deal with similar situations, with successful and reasonably easy outcomes. I was in the office, as was our new intern, Emily when the call came in and as I was the most easily available vet, it was decided I would go and take Emily with me. This is a situation she would have to deal with on her own when more experienced, here was a chance to learn!

The journey there would take us about forty minutes and on arriving on the farm Anthony greeted us somewhat concerned with the state of his cow. As with the previous cases I had been to here, the cow had been fed on potatoes along with her mates, but she had taken one too big to swallow whole. She had tried and it was now stuck somewhere between her mouth and her rumen. With this blockage, it meant that she could not eructate, burp, so she had gas building up in her rumen, a by-product of her digestive processes in this stomach. This was somewhat obvious as her left side was becoming more and more enlarged, and she was in some discomfort and distress.

The standard equipment in these cases is after securing the cow, a halter, a gag and a stomach tube. The gag fits neatly into the angles of the jaw, having large grooves top and bottom which fit over the rows of molar teeth. When inserting it into the cow's mouth one invariably has to grab the cow's tongue, pulling it out and to the opposite side that you are going to insert the gag before sliding into over the teeth and as far into the mouth as one can. With that done, the cow cannot close her mouth and more importantly bite you or anything you may place in her mouth. Once this is done you can examine inside the mouth and if necessary, insert a stomach tube down over the back of her tongue and into her oesophagus. For cases like this , there is a more rigid stomach tube called a Probang which has a narrow canal running through it which can accommodate a strong plastic probe long enough to extend beyond the end of the tube, but at the mouth end having a small circular handle that can be used to slide the probe backwards and forwards within the tube. If any blockage, or in the case of "blown" cows, is easily removed then a larger bore tube can be used to release any gas from the rumen more quickly.

We got Anthony's cow into his cattle crush, a squeeze as she was already distending in her flanks and from a quick examination, I could point out to Emily a point just anterior to the thoracic inlet where I could feel a large foreign body in the cow's oesophagus. It almost certainly was a potato and was stuck at a delicate part, if we were too forceful in trying to remove it, trying to push it on further down, there would be the risk of rupturing her oesophagus and that would invariably be fatal.

This didn't look as if it was going to be easy and as the cow was getting more and more distressed our first decision was made in that we should release the gas building up in her rumen, a relatively simple procedure of placing a canula through her flank and into the rumen, immediately letting the gas out. You all will have heard the tales of attendants smoking while this procedure is carried out, and of course the gases building up, methane, are highly inflammable. Need I say more, other than that was not going to happen in this case. They now make these wonderful cannulas called *Red Devil's* that screw into the rumen through the abdominal musculature so they will stay in place until removed.

The cow was instantly more comfortable, now all we would have to do was to try and get the potato to go one way or the other past this narrowing stopping its passage into the rumen. I hoped this would be a simple as the last couple I had dealt with here.

Had not I somewhere along the line in the past suggested

chopping these bigger spuds up with a spade so that this could not happen, I knew I must have but it didn't always happen. Now was the time to roll up our sleeves and get to work on the problem at hand.

I found that by squeezing behind the potato through the skin it was possible to move it slightly upwards, but not far. Next would be to try passing a stomach tube down her throat and see if we could move the potato the other way at all. That would mean putting the gag in her mouth, I could demonstrate that to by student.

It was time to roll my sleeves up and with a waterproof top on and get down to the serious business of trying to help this cow with her difficulties. First, I slid the gag down the left side of her mouth, making sure it was firmly wedged between her upper and lower sets of molars. Happy with that, I gently inserted the Probang into her mouth, over the back of her tongue and then as she swallowed, slipping gently into and down her oesophagus. Down it went inch by inch, until we reached the point where the potato was stuck. Resistance, it was going to go no further. I would try a few gentle taps, sliding the Probang backwards and forwards, tap, tap on the potato so as not to be too forceful and create more problems. It was not going to budge.

If it was not going to go down, it was going to have to come up. How could we manage that, we had already managed to manipulate it up the oesophagus a little from outside with our hands. I withdrew the Probang, and we decided that if Emily tried to move the potato up, then I would try and reach down the cow's throat and see if I could get hold of it and bring it back up into the mouth and out.

I gently inserted my hand, arm into her mouth and then down her throat and into her oesophagus. With all my winter clothing on I found that my arm was too big with sleeves of shirt and jumper rolled up under my protective top. Also, being a big cow, I was not tall enough.

I asked Anthony to get me a bale of straw to stand on while

I stripped off top the waist, replacing my waterproof top over my now naked torso, it was too cold to be dressed like this.

We were ready to try again! Standing on my bale, I reached down again. I may be vertically challenged, but I do have long arms and now without the impediment of rolled up sleeves I could now reach into the cow's oesophagus and with Emily gently trying to press the potato upwards, we attempted to get down to it again. How frustrating, I could reach it with my fingertips, but could I get my fingers around it, no I could not. If only Emily could just manoeuvre the damn thing up just a couple of inches perhaps then I would be successful. But she could not, and we struggled for a few minutes with my arm down the cow's throat without success. She, of course, did not take too kindly to be having someone's arm down her throat, I probably would have felt the same. She struggled to remove herself from this situation, throwing her head from side to side, me of course going with her, she was stronger than me and I had my arm well down inside her. It was a fight and tiring for me, resisting her and with one arm otherwise engaged.

We decided we would swop over, perhaps I could manage to get the potato a little further up than Emily and with her smaller hand she may be able to reach around it and pull it up. Obviously, we did not ask her to strip to the waist and hopefully with narrower arms she may succeed where I hadn't. It was worth a try!

We swopped, I tried to manoeuvre the potato up, and it did move though whether it was actually moving up or just the oesophagus being stretched upwards I didn't know. Emily stood on the bale and tried to reach down, but her arms were not as long as mine, she couldn't even reach the potato. We would have to swop back again so I held the offending thing where I had moved it up to until Emily could grip it there herself. Then for me it was back onto the bale and putting my arm back into the cow's mouth, I reached down once again.

Yes, we had made a little progress as I could now feel more but there was an increasing amount of saliva collecting making any grip more and more difficult, especially as it was still at the tips of my fingers.

I struggled on and to be honest was making no progress, with the cow offering increased resistance to this insult I was inflicting on her. As she spung her head from side to side, my arm would come increasingly in contact with her teeth and was getting more and more scratched. I was also getting quite tired.

We had reached a point where we could not move the potato one way or the other. I was worried about causing an acute oesophagitis or rupturing it completely. Options we had were to do surgery and try and remove the potato, dissecting down onto it but this could be fraught with danger due to its position so near to the chest and with so many vital structures running close by, vagal nerves, carotid arteries to name two.

We decided that we would see if we could damage the potato's surface more with the Probang so that the cow's digestive juices could work on it and aid its digestion so that it could pass on in time. With the canula in her side, in her rumen, she could not blow up with gas again, I hoped in a short time that natural digestion would get the cow out of her predicament.

With the probe inside the Probang, again I inserted it into the cow and banged gently against the potato with it. I could feel its edges increasingly roughened. That was all that we could do, removing the gag, giving the cow a drug that may relax the muscles around the potato and make her feel a little more comfortable.

We washed up, cleaned our equipment, and said we would ring in the morning to see how the cow was and if there was any more we could do.

Getting redressed, I realised how much my arm had been "damaged" with multiple teeth scratches all over it, my right arm. Over the next twenty-four hours I could see and feel more and more damage under my skin, areas of hardness developing as more and more inflammation took place.

I rang Anthony the following morning, good news. The cow seemed far more comfortable and was now drinking and if she was doing that then there could be no obstruction into her stomach, the potato had moved. Which way, up or down I would never know but good news and with antibiotic cover, she would make a complete recovery.

My arm, the thickening under the skin would take some weeks to heal, the scarring on my skin, it took months before they all finally went away.

And from all these traumas, we never had to go to a potato choke on the farm again. A lesson learned, he made sure all feed potatoes were chopped so easy to masticate and to swallow. But again, something so easy to avoid.

A bruised and chewed arm for me, the cow, at last managing to get the potato where it could be digested, but I guess I can sympathise with her despite the state of my arm at the time. My experiences of having an endoscope put down my throat was not one of my greatest, gagging constantly until they gave me something to sedate me to allow the doctors to carry out their procedures, if it were an arm, heaven forbid how I would have felt, whether there was anything stuck there or not.

I suppose in my early days I was quite apprehensive about passing a stomach tube down a cow's throat, worrying whether I had got it down the oesophagus or the windpipe, but with experience and having confidence after a while that my gag was firmly in place, it became a piece of cake. I have spoken before in *"The Quiet Vet"* about what a great introduction it was when a stomach pump was invented to get fluids into cows quickly rather than the painstakingly intravenous injections. The volumes needed to get into a dehydrated cow are huge and if not given slowly into the blood stream can soon overload the system risking pulmonary oedema and drowning the cow while trying to save her. By mouth, twenty, thirty litres of made up solutions suitable to what you were trying to treat could be administered within minutes, the only energy exerted being after when you have inserted the tube down the cow's throat into the rumen, you have to pump the fluid from buckets down her throat. Exercise for one arm and not that tiring. A few years ago, this used to be a vet only procedure but now farmers and herdsmen have become proficient enough themselves to do this and our only involvement can be servicing the pumps, everything has a limited shelf life.

They have become more than competent at using these pumps for routine conditions, as a pick-me up after calving or surgery as a follow up treatment, energy drenches, drenches to restore acid-base balance in the rumen and more. But it is something that us as vets still do on a regular basis especially in extremely sick and toxic cows e.g., those that have an acute E. coli mastitis, sometimes administering it at the same time as giving hypertonic saline intravenous fluids so that fluids in the stomach are absorbed more quickly. This use of fluid therapy in cattle medicine has been a life saver.

But I can recall in my not-too-distant past where one farm manager got it wrong! I had examined his cow and had said there was need for fluids to be given. My trusty assistant, the farm manager, wanted to show how competent he was, there was no way he was going to let me, the vet, give the fluids. He assured me he was more than competent to do it himself and having got his buckets ready of fluids, secured the cow and passed the stomach pump himself. Having passed it he listened to the end of the pump and was positive there were no breaths coming up through it, just a ruminal smell. He was not even going to let me check, he soon had the other end of the pump in the fluids and was pumping merrily away. I didn't have his confidence and despite asking him to be sure (I guess I always had a feeling that I had the tube where it should be and if not happy would withdraw it and start again until happy) he carried on with a smirk on his face that he was showing the vet how good he was. The cow did not look happy, something was wrong, I was sure he was not in the rumen but had passed it down the trachea and when the cow started coughing, it confirmed my suspicions. It took a lot of persuading to get him to stop but at last he did. Alas it was too late for the cow whose lungs were now full of the contents of his bucket, she was drowning.

A little fluid the lungs may cope with, an aspiration

pneumonia is always a risk in cattle when drenching, or when they are recumbent inhaling their own ruminal contents. But this volume and with the powders mixed into it, there was no way she was going to survive this. He withdrew the tube from her, but it was too late, she sunk to her knees and that was that.

He had in all probability drenched many cows in the past successfully, was he just unlucky this time in wanting to show off in front of me. Lessons learned, I made sure I always did the job myself or supervised the cowman if he was doing it, making sure that both he and I were sure and happy the stomach tube should be where it was.

Of course, the old way of drenching cattle was with a wine bottle, the shape of a Reisling bottle being ideal to get over that lump at the base of the tongue and down her throat. Drenching of course usually meant mixing some powders in water and then thrusting it down the cow's throat, and as she swallowed the bottle emptied taking its contents down into the stomach. Some of those drenches smelt, probably tasted okay, others smelled vile, and you could appreciate the cow's struggle trying not to swallow these horrible liquids. How many times all those years ago, especially when cows were smaller had you emptied the bottle and remover it from the cow's mouth only for her then to try and cough it all back up again, mostly over me! Then there were others that smelled of aniseed, a smell I love, and as the cow gulped happily away as this went down her, I would be quite envious of her having this aniseed drink. Bring me a Sambuca!

There were other times when things did not go quite right. Those conditions where you were not sure whether there were nerve problems as well, especially if it is affecting the vagus nerve. Conditions like tetanus, lock jaw, affect the nerves and though more generally bloat being a symptom in cattle as the cow cannot eructate, if her jaws are clamped then it is very difficult to "tube" her. When you are sure of your diagnosis then welfare comes into play, and it is kinder to have the animal euthanised. Cows with Listeriosis can also have facial nerve deficits, and the vagus is one of those. Though more usually showing facial signs, a dropped ear on onside, a drooping eyelid, circling, lesions affecting one side of the brain, I can remember one cow that it also affected her rumen and ability to swallow. A lot of cases if one catches them early enough can respond to treatment, antibiotics and supportive treatment, but this particular cow did need fluids as she couldn't drink. Tim, the farmer and I decided we would have to stomach pump fluids into her and so me, having managed to get the tube down her we proceeded to get twenty-five litres down the tube. That should aid her recovery, or so we thought. Having finished, we slowly withdrew the tube back out through her mouth, job done. Following the tube out came the twenty-five litres of liquid, may be not all of it but certainly enough to shower me and Tim standing behind me.

The joys of farm animal medicine!

You can get just as messy whichever end of the cow on which you are working. Perhaps I finish at the right time as cows get bigger and bigger and it becomes more of a struggle for a little chap like me to wrestle with them, drenching or tubing them. But through the years it has given many laughs, and more than a few bruises!

LORD OF THE RINGS:

I HAVE SPOKEN before about vets and their great ability to loose things, or more likely to have misplaced equipment while on farm, and then another of us colleagues having to retrieve said bit of apparatus when either the vet owner has found a need for his own equipment, or more likely, a farmer ringing up to say that the vet had left something on his farm. We did have one or two vets in the practice who were especially adept at this, and one or two of us who always seemed to be the ones who had to do the retrieval. There is nothing more frustrating than getting organized to do a job and finding the essential piece of kit needed for that job had gone missing, either left on the farm by the previous user, or still in that vet's car. Much time was wasted sorting this out, retrieving equipment to conduct the next task.

If I were never that guilty of this, other than leaving the odd stethoscope here and there, usually hung over a gate while I was examining a cow or calf further, I did always carry two spares in the car so was never without until reunited with number one, my favourite one.

However, for those who have read my previous exploits, they will know that my failings invariably involved hearing aids, and much to my cost. I did in the end invent a method that would ensure their safeguard, saving time on those fruitless searches I had had in the past.

I had moved on to more expensive losses. For those many years of my first marriage I had never worn, never wanted a wedding ring. I always thought it pointless to have a ring that I would be

99

taking off and putting back on every five minutes, sooner or later I would either forget to take it off and find while calving a cow it was still on me and causing a little discomfort, or I would lose it. I could have had a chain around my neck with it on, but I never really fancied that idea either. So, for years I never wore a ring.

Second time around, I thought "why not", I have bought enough for other people so why should not I have one as well, and it was there as a token of love. So, on that delightful day in 2017 at Shrewsbury Castle, Jane and I did exchange rings, plain, amazingly simple, and similar in white gold. And there it proudly rested on the appropriate finger of my left hand, unless I was working when arriving on a farm, I would take it off and place it carefully in my waistcoat pocket until my jobs were completed when it would be placed back on my finger again. In the summer months when it was warm enough that the waistcoat body warmer was not needed, then I placed the ring in the well behind my car's gear stick for safe keeping.

And that system remained in place for many weeks, a routine was established which seemed to work well without me misplacing the ring, nor some cow having this piece of metal shoved up their backside on a vet's finger. That experience was not that comfortable for the vet and his finger either.

So, after eighteen months of my second marriage, and having become well accustomed to the wearing of a ring for the first time in my life, I set off for my fortnightly routine visit at Binweston on a chilly late winter's morning. I arrived in the yard, slightly early as usual and prepared to get ready for the visit, starting with taking off the ring and placing it in the left-hand pocket. Then it was time to get my kit on, boots and protective clothing and then getting the drugs and equipment I would need for the visit, taking it to the station by the cattle crush where we operated from, and waited for Fiona and Gwyn to arrive. This is a big herd, milking in excess of nine hundred cows in two calving blocks, so at this time of year it would not be uncommon to see fifty plus cows on a morning visit, post-calving checks and any non-bullers (cows which had not been seen bulling to be served again).

So, it would be nearly two hours before I returned to the car again after cleaning off my protective clothing, putting my equipment back into the car and preparing to leave. I would have to admit after a busy morning that the last thing on my mind was my wedding ring as I set off from the farm, ringing into the office to say I had finished and was heading off to my next call.

It would be later when I had finished my morning round that my hand delved back into my waistcoat pocket to retrieve my ring and replace it back on my finger.

It was not there!

Where could it be? I got out of the car, checked the pocket again, then all my other pockets and the well behind the gearstick. Nothing!

Had I got it wrong and taken it off by the cattle crush and put it in my drugs tray? I did not think I had but worth checking so that was what I duly did next, but still nothing.

I rang Fiona at lunchtime and told her I had mislaid my ring, could she just have a quick glance around where my car was and around the table where I had had my drugs tray just in case I had mislaid it there. I could not think where else it could be.

I returned home to Jane that evening ringless.

Do I tell her or wait and see what crops up when I had spoken to Fiona again? She and Gwyn had turned the place upside down looking but nothing. I had searched the car again but nothing on that count either, it was a lost cause.

Still the question, should I tell Jane? I was grateful for the effort those at Binweston had put into trying to find the ring and gave my sincere thanks next time I was there.

"What did Jane say?" they asked.

"I have not told her yet that her token of love has been mislaid. I have checked on Amazon and have managed to find an identical replacement, it is on its way. And a third of the price of the one Jane had bought me from the jewellers!" I said.

By the next time I was at Binweston, I had a wedding ring

again. And Jane had not noticed its' absence. All was well!

The weeks passed into early spring and on one sunny afternoon I was called to Strawberry Fields to see a sick calf. The usual routine as I got out of the car, stethoscope in hand and set off across the newly bedded straw yard to find the calf I needed to examine. Ring off and into my waistcoat pocket, find the calf, take its temperature then listen to its chest, examine its navel, and then treat it with what I thought were the appropriate drugs. I washed off and returned to the car, reaching into my pocket to return my betrothal ring back to its designated finger.

Nothing!

Not again, it could not be more than eight weeks since the last one had gone, and now again! Perhaps this wedding ring idea was not one of my best. I looked at the freshly bedded yard and thought "no way" am I going to find it in there. I did tell Dorian and his daughter but knew in my heart of hearts that there was not even any point in looking, it would really have been looking for a ring in a haystack!

Strawberry Fields forever. I do not think so!

And.......

I would have to tell Jane this time. And would I now have to get a third ring, pennies were a little tight!

I did tell her, and she appreciated it was just one of those things. One day, there was no hurry, I would get another ring. Good old Amazon!

But it did seem strange after wearing a ring for those first few months of wedded bliss to be ringless again, my finger felt bare.

Every now and again a vet's car needs a good clean out, a wash (though with me, never one of my fortes, I think I just move the mud around to different locations on the car), clear the back seat and give a good hoover around. Sweeping around under the driver's seat in Vectra number two, what was that I just felt. I ran my hand around under the seat again and.... pulled out a ring, a wedding ring.

And it was one of mine.

I rolled it around between my fingers, it looked no worse for wear other than a little tarnished. I placed it back on my finger, relief that I had found one.

But which one was it? I suspect it was actually the ring placed on my finger at my wedding but could not be one hundred percent sure. Never mind, I had a ring again, I was pleased.

And Jane was pleased too!

There may have been one or two more mishaps from then until retirement, but mainly in the garden when I had been weeding or planting perennials, rummaging around in the soil with my hands to establish the plant in its new position. But I had always realised the ring had come off and readily found it straight away.

The ring lasted me until retirement and beyond. What I did find after finishing work was that I had lost weight and some days the ring was a very loose fit on my finger, sometimes it could easily fall off by itself. But all was good, I was always aware that it had slipped off and was able to retrieve it instantly.

Yes, I did do the odd vet job after retirement and when I knew I was doing something in the line of vetting, now that I would arrive in my best car, my Qashqai as the Vectra had long gone, I would meticulously place ring in the mug wells for safe keeping, usually before I had arrived on the farm, and replace it back onto my finger when back in the car and driving off.

However, some months later, in the spring of 2022 I had visited my Financial Advisor in Wolverhampton on a warm, beautifully sunny day. It was approaching lunchtime; I had just got back into the car to head home on the M54 when I got a call from Bob just outside Newport. He had a cow calving and needed assistance. I would have to divert off the motorway and make my way to the farm, I told him I would be about twenty-five minutes. I was not dressed to calve a cow, but hoped the protective clothing I had with me would keep me in good stead, nice and clean. It was ten minutes or so before I arrived on the farm that I removed the ring and placed it in its resting place.

A successful calving followed my arrival, and I managed to

stay fairly clean. Cow and the new arrival calf were returned to a loose box to become acquainted with each other and for the calf to receive its colostrum from mum, so important in its first few hours of life to protect against disease.

I cleaned up, I was done and got ready to drive home for that long-awaited lunch. While driving I reached down to retrieve my ring and put it back on my finger. But it was not there. Not again! I got home and searched the car thoroughly but unsuccessfully, the ring had disappeared again, it was jinxed.

With no success, I rang Bob up and told him of my mishap. It was unlikely but I suppose there was a slight chance it may be lying around where I had parked my car, but I did not hold out much hope. I heard nothing from Bob so assumed it was gone. He was highly amused about the mishaps of said ring but no news, then no ring. I was there again a couple of days later for another calving but could see no sign myself either.

It was a week later that Bob rang me with the news that his helper, another Bob, had found my ring.

But he said, "It may not look quite the same as the last time I had seen it"!

"I would collect it next time I was on the farm," I said.

My next visit, when we were finished, Bob retrieved the ring from the house and have it back into my grateful hand. Indeed, it was a different ring, now very misshapen and with very rough edges. I could still get it on, and it certainly did not feel as mobile on my finger now, mainly because of its changed shape, it now having a sort of flat side.

I managed to file some of the rough edges down with a metal nail file, I would have to take it to a jeweller some time to see if its shape could be restored. Something for another day.

There may have been the odd mishap after that, once losing it in the garden again and resorting to using Jane's metal detector to track it down. I had been potting tubs and filling them up with compost, rather than emptying every pot of plants and compost it would be easier to use the detector to find which contained the gold treasure. Both Jane and I tried on different occasions the following morning, but with no success, I eventually found it in front of one of my raised borders I had been working on, just sitting in the grass.

Four or five months later, Chris asked me if I could look at a sick cow for him. She was struggling to stand and walk in from the field. It was only a couple of miles from home, but I did have commitments that morning so said I would call in when he had got back from his lunch. When I arrived, he was getting the cows in for afternoon milking, but this cow was not interested in following her mates, she had remained lying down in the field some way away.

I gathered up what I thought I would need to examine her, and we set off down the track to the field she was in. When there I put on some rubber gloves, remembering then that I had not taken the ring off. Never mind, thinking I could feel it under the glove, I was not going to lose it from under this. A rectal examination may be slightly uncomfortable but never mind.

The cow was not good, I did not hold out much chance for her survival, but we gave her pain relief, offered her some water and would have to see what the morning would bring.

We returned to Chris's truck and started to head back towards the farm. I went to take the gloves off and thought, strange, I cannot feel a ring there. I removed the left glove carefully, and no, there was no ring. I told Chris, we stopped the truck, I checked my tray I had taken my equipment in, and Chris rooted around the back seat which one would have to be honest, was a mess. Wire, bags, tools, fence posts, they were all there! Nothing, so we reversed back to the paddock where we had looked at the cow, walked across to where she was and had a quick search. Having had so little rain for weeks, the pasture was fairly bare, dry and hard. There was only a small area the ring could possibly be in, and a quick glance around revealed nothing. I was aware I was holding the milking up so I told Chris not to worry, I would return in the morning with Jane's metal detector.

I got home and checked by box again, and all my pockets,

the discarded gloves but no luck, the ring was definitely missing. I told Jane it had gone AWOL again, what did she expect! But she was excited about using her metal detector again and for a useful purpose, she said she would come with me in the morning.

That was that for the day, we would see what tomorrow would bring.

Why the worry of wearing a ring while doing my job? Firstly, there was the risk of it coming off while doing a calving or lambing, losing it inside the animal creating a foreign body which may or not be expelled at a later date. Secondly, it was uncomfortable, even painful when carrying out a rectal examination as the ring was pressed down your finger and down to where it joins the rest of the hand. Finally, I have heard of many sleeving injuries, and Chris had told me that he had received one when the ring had caught on something and had cut down deep into the finger, removing a large proportion of skin. Very painful and something that takes a long time to heal.

Later that evening, Jane retired to bed before me.

"Come up here now," she shouted down the stairs so I could hear. "You need to see this, and I won't be coming with you in the morning with my metal detector."

I climbed the stairs to be greeted by Jane holding my ring in her fingers.

"Where did you find that?" I asked.

"I pulled back the sheet on the bed and there it was lying on the bottom sheet," she replied.

It had slipped off my finger the previous night while in bed, I had never had it on all day! But why did I think that I had felt it under my glove in the truck? That will be a mystery.

I rang Chris in the morning to tell him my embarrassing news and had hoped he had not wasted any more time on a fruitless search. He told me that the farmer's son was just about to go up to the field and check the area we had marked the previous day with a small stick. He too had a metal detector.

However, Chris told me he had done a complete search of

the truck again, which was not a complete waste of time as he had taken everything out of it, and it had had a long overdue tidy up.

The result was so unlikely and amusing, he just laughed.

Will I get a chain to put the ring on around my neck, or just carry on losing it from time to time. It has lived a very charmed life.

A tale that certainly has a ring to it!

POLITICS AND THINGS:

A S I WRITE we seem to be in a time of crisis. Post Brexit whether you believed it to be right or wrong, we now have a cost-of-living crisis, immigration, and a war in Europe. Food shortages in certain products, strikes causing disruption to everyday life and of course the ever-eternal threat of climate change continues to worry us along with an energy crisis with soaring prices for a basic necessity of life during our cold winters. Is everything going wrong, sometimes it seems as if it is! As I write, the heavens have opened once again over the past few days, all that Welsh rain is now hurtling into the Severn and Dee valleys and as is the norm these past few years, Shropshire and Cheshire with Worcestershire and Gloucestershire to follow, we are in flood. Up go the flood barriers in both Shrewsbury and Ironbridge, how many times has that happened over the past two or three years. The effects of climate change or are we just going through a period of warmer and wetter winters.

There seems much change, a lot of disruption, a lot of unrest at this present time. We have come out of the Covid pandemic though it still rages in the background, but we do not worry so much about it now into the turmoil that months of lockdown, furlough and all the economic implications that were caused by one little mutating virus. But all those other troubles mentioned above have now exacerbated everyone's state of mind and the country, Europe, is all doom and gloom.

I have a very positive outlook on life these days having recovered from depression those ten long years ago, and now should be my, Jane and my time as we start our retirement and look forward to a well-earned rest, relaxation and the chance to do and see those things we have craved for during our working career. Despite the doom and gloom around us, I still maintain that attitude. I do not want to go back to where I was in my dark years, those years which I struggled through and struggled for so long to get out of. I will have a better future, remaining positive even if all around are not, enjoying life and enjoying the wonderful surrounds I have, the countryside and its wildlife. What joy it gives me to watch in the garden now the visitors that now attend my recently put-up bird feeder. My garden, for so long the habitat of a pair of nesting blackbirds and the ever-present pigeons and scavenging jackdaws, but now visited by sparrows, wrens, robins, coal its, long tailed tits, bluetits and for ultimate joy, nuthatches. Nature can be so enlightening and consuming.

But what does this all have to do with my veterinary career and its future, and the future of farming in this country?

I guess this is the time to state that what I write now is my opinion and my opinion alone, though I guess there may be many who would share the same sentiments.

We live in a beautiful country, Wales and Scotland are likewise. I have never visited Northern Ireland so cannot comment on there, but even a spawling conurbation like Telford where I live has its special places. The Town Park, the Wrekin to mention a couple where nature still thrives. But there is a constant challenge now between town and country, needs for housing and the rural landscape. The environmental activist, Greta Thunberg, in her rallying calls has blamed my and past generations for the state and future of the world, wanting actions to preserve something for her generation and the next, putting a halt to climate change, increasing levels of greenhouse gases so that life as we know it can be maintained. But as I walk around my locality, a common past time for me now, how many food wrappers from fast food outlets, McDonald's, KFC, pizza places do I see chucked out of cars, lying around in hedgerows, on pavements etc and this is the food of her generation. None of us respect our environment enough, though giving a little praise where it is due, many farmers try to.

We have a rising population in this country from increased birth rates, us living longer, immigration and a refugee problem that no-one seems to have got to grips with. So, to me, there are two basic necessities going forward, enough housing and enough food. I guess the reason I voted for Brexit was mainly because I hoped politicians would grasp the concept that we in this country could produce a lot more food of our own, being far more self-sufficient and offering a greater degree of food security. I hoped with some sort of co-ordination and without offering huge subsidies, that we could produce and not import, be far more reliant on our own producers to feed the nation. And hopefully in doing that, a bonus would be that it would create a lot more jobs. Now I am disappointed.

But with that, we have also had to look at alternative forms of green energy. With the expanding population, energy requirements increase as does the need for housing. Brown belts get built on; green belts follow slowly meaning there is less land for producing food.

I suppose all those years ago, the two main reasons I wanted to become a vet were a love of the countryside and farming, and a chance to help in the food production of this land, essentially that is what farming is about, producing food to feed the nation. That is whether it is producing feed or managing grassland to feed animals to produce, or directly producing food from crops. Whether meat eaters, vegans, or vegetarians, we need land to produce food, and in the livestock industry then that is where my role came in as a vet, keeping the livestock I cared for healthy and productive by preventing or treating disease.

I suppose one of my pet hates now is seeing the vast acreage that is now getting covered with solar panels. Yes, it is a green energy, but I feel it is wrong that so much good land is taken up with these. I have always thought that wind turbines are a form of ugly beauty, one of the things I look out for on my walking trips to the Lake District is when the M6 crosses Shap Fell and these giants emerge over the hill side. Even in a barren landscape like that they do not look out of place in my mind, and they are using one of nature's resources while the land around them can still be used. More importantly they do produce a great deal of energy, tapping a natural resource, the wind. Jane and my ever more frequent visits to the north coast of Wales, looking out to sea from Llandudno and seeing a vast field of these turbines. To me they do not look out of place and supply power to hundreds of homes. Off the coast of Norfolk in the North Sea likewise. Areas of moorland could also be used, supplying a better local economy to these poorer areas. There is so much potential for utilising this resource to the full, as well as having a large coastline where the tide comes in and out every day, another natural resource, wave power. There is so much potential for us to again be self-sufficient with something we already have in abundance, and with our already commissioned nuclear power stations our dependence on fossil fuels would be diminished, even unnecessary except for running vehicles.

But to me solar energy is a waste of land which could be better used for food production, whether that be livestock farming or cereal production. I was driving up the M1 in Northamptonshire not so long ago and was horrified the acreage in the distance covered with these things, land which could be used to produce food. To me, every building has a roof. Agricultural and industrial buildings have vast roofs, and this is where solar panels should be. With the price of energy these days, and from what some farmers have told me of how much their energy costs have risen this year, an investment in these panels on their own roofs would reap benefits after a while, probably also producing an excess of energy that can go into the National Grid. To me, any new building on a farm, on an industrial site should have solar panels. I would add to that, any new build housing estate, is it going to put that much on the asking price if panels were put on their roofs, benefitting the occupants in providing some of their own energy and reducing their bills. There would be no need to give subsidies to householders for installing the panels, they would already be there and included in the asking price with the incoming householder about to benefit straight away from their investment.

There is so much potential available as a natural resource and it seems a shame to me not to be using this, it to me just requires a little thought and investment to come up with such simple solutions that are more environmentally friendly.

But where does this fit in with my views of farming and my career as a vet. I suppose it does not other than my personal wish that we should be more food self-sufficient in this country, and more energy sufficient without having to resort to the use of fossil fuels. We manage our natural resources well which means using the land to grow food, and other natural resources to produce energy. This is a personal opinion I must stress again.

But farmers do find other energy sources. Maize is grown in abundance in those parts of the country where the climate is suitable, both as a fodder crop for cattle feed, being a rich source of energy to produce high yields of milk from, and also as a "feeder" of digesters, being fed into them to produce energy suitable for use as a power source. On my visits to Africa, it has horrified those Indigenous peoples whose basic diet is based around maize that we both feed it to cattle and use it as an energy source. I suppose it worries me a bit that it goes into digesters when it could be fed to cattle. It is the cob which is the rich energy source for nutrition so there is so much of the plant which is of little value, but at least chopped finely in maize silage, it firstly adds bulk to the feed, and secondly dilutes the rich energy cobs meaning that the rumen can make better use of the raw material, if the cobs were digested too quickly, it would soon create a very acidic rumen and the health of the cow would suffer. On my travels in East Africa, I have tried to find a use for the stems, the dried leaves, the low energy part of the plant which does not go for human consumption, discussing it with local small holders without finding a solution. When fodder is short, especially in the dry season, it seems a shame we cannot us it somehow.

Biodigesters do offer a source of producing energy and would be classed as a 100% renewable (no carbon) process. They offer the chance to turn low-grade organic waste into a high-value energy source where bacteria anaerobically digest this organic material into "Biogas", a mixture of Methane, carbon Dioxide and Hydrogen Sulphide, similar in proportion to that of Natural Gas. A chemical energy is produced which is combustible and releases energy when burnt which can be used to generate electricity or other fuels. It has its advantages in being permanently available, transportable, and storable. Furthermore, its waste product, the digestate is a good source of fertiliser that can be used to return vital nutrients to the soil.

If I think it is a waste of a feeding material such as maize to us in this process, then certainly some of the bigger dairy producers and large chicken units are now installing these digester plants onto their farms as a way of getting energy but also a way of using the vast amounts of waste they produce in the form of manure. The downside is the expense of installing these plants, but I am sure that those large units will overtime pay easily pay for their investment and be offering a greener future. The high humus content of the digestate, as well as its high fertiliser value will greatly enhance the soil structure when it is applied to the land. So here I think, there is a double bonus but only affordable by some.

We have to produce more food with our ever-expanding population, our resources become more limited with the increasing need for housing, and for leisure. This is not just a problem for us but is a worldwide issue, but our problem is that we are only a small island and so our population density is high. We have t balance the needs of that increasing population with our ability to produce food, we cannot rely on importing everything as other countries endure the same problems. The Brazilian rainforests disappear as more and more forests are reclaimed to grow soya, a rich plant protein source and widely used in animal feeds. There is no return of goodness to this soil, it becomes barren, more forest is reclaimed and the effects on greenhouse gases we all know about.

So, to me it is vital we use our land well, and respect it. I recently visited a farm where he was processing his manure, dividing a liquid part which was rich in nitrogen and a more solid part containing potash and phosphates. In doing this, he was more able to try and supply his grasslands with the essential nutrients they need when they need it. He was producing his own fertiliser, and of course there are costs involved in doing this but when one weighs that up with the spiralling costs of artificial fertilisers, something greatly affected by the war in Ukraine where so much originates from, then he can maintain productivity while keeping some handle on his costs. Other farmers to reduce their costs have just cut back on fertilizer use, meaning their grasslands are not so productive and they either have to accept reduced yields or supplement feed in another form, again not cheap. If there is less productivity from our land, then to produce the same, we need more of it, again the challenge of how we can best use our natural resources.

Methane has come up in the conversation when talking about digesters and somewhere one has to mention that and its effect on global warming. Both methane and carbon dioxide gases are produced in this digester process but here the gases are trapped. Of far more significance are the greenhouse gases produced in nature. Deforestation affects the absorption of carbon dioxide from the atmosphere as plants play a part in this process, and that is where the loss of such as the Amazon rainforests has a significant affect with its effect on destroying the protective ozone layer and the ability of them to absorb heat from the sun. Without them the world would be a very cold place, but as their levels rise in the atmosphere then the temperatures on Earth continue to rise and at their present rate, towards worrying levels. A small rise would probably increase productivity of crops, making some areas warmer and so more productive in say growing maize, or even soya where it is not grown now. But further rises would have deleterious effects, being too hot for crop production causing dramatic shifts in our climate.

I am no expert on all this but even over the past few years in Shropshire we have seen such changes, milder winters with the Severn flooding more frequently. Ironbridge and Shrewsbury have suffered time after time, and that iconic view I have of the Wrekin and Shropshire Plain from the bridge at Atcham is often in winter now one of a watery landscape. Warmer, dry summers like the one experienced just gone in 2022 where temperatures rose and were sustained in the high twenties centigrade with days and days without rain.

The effects on farming, heat stress in cattle especially and of course the reduction in crop productivity meaning poorer cereal yields and reduced milk production in dairy cows unless feed is supplemented, either from conservation crops providing winter forage (silage) or the increased use of concentrate feeds which are very expensive and ultimately will push the price up to the consumer. Certainly in 2022 there were some burnt grasslands, winter forage had to be used in late June and July, there was no grass to cut for hay and winter food supplies were depleted.

But why does this affect us as farmers and vets. The poor old cow seems to get blamed so much these days because she eats grass, it enters her stomach, her rumen, and then is regurgitated to be chewed over and over again to get more value from the feed. Rumination, and it produces methane. The cow gets blamed, but what about all the other ruminants, not just in this country but worldwide. Those millions of sheep grazing hear and especially on uplands where the land cannot be used for anything else. Big dairy producing countries like New Zealand, the massive ranches in the States, in South America and we must not forget those huge populations of ruminants wandering the savannahs of East Africa, nor those herdsmen whose livestock sustain a living for them. Do they have a significant effect on climate change, this is not for me to say, I don't know enough about it, but compared with cars, planes and industry, surely not!

We hear more and more about a push to going vegan or vegetarian as these livestock get blamed for more and more, but we all have a right to choose what we eat, are we not omnivores? And of course, livestock produce one very important commodity as a by-product from their main production and that comes out of their rear ends. If we have talked about digestate being a rich source of fertiliser and humus to improve soil structure, then so does manure, whether from cattle, sheep, pigs, or poultry. In my visits to Africa and especially when working, teaching for the charity *Send a Cow (now Ripple Effect)* I have seen how important the conservation of these waste products are in improving soil quality and then being able to produce more productive crops to improve the nutrition of small holders starting out on these projects. Greater production has allowed an increase in family wealth, health and then education, and the ripple effect of others seeing these benefits has been the plus, spreading the word and in time giving more and more people a better life.

Is there a plus on the horizon. In New Zealand there has been a project to produce a sustained release methane inhibitor technology for grass-fed animals, backed by several million dollars of state aid with the hope that a commercially viable bolus can be produced by 2025 that will deliver at least a seventy percent reduction in ruminant animals' methane emissions over six months.

The slow-release bolus will deliver a methane inhibitor at the site of methane production, in the rumen. As far as the company's initial trials have gone, they have achieved a ninety percent methane reduction over an eighty-day period, a positive result although the aim would be to extend that period to seventy percent over six months.

Certainly, in New Zealand it is thought some fifty percent of greenhouse gases come from agriculture with three quarters of this coming from methane produced by ruminants. Other countries are looking at in-feed additives to achieve some sort of methane emission reduction, in New Zealand where livestock production tends to be a grass-fed system then boluses rather than feed additives offer a far more practical solution. With this development, in New Zealand they hope to achieve by 2030 their target of a ten percent reduction in 2017 levels.

Time will tell how successful this will be, but it is a positive step in the right direction certainly in a country that is so dependent on agriculture for its economic survival. And if similar research and development is taking place elsewhere and similar results can be achieved, then it offers a lot of hope for livestock production to continue and not be continually slated for its methane production.

I guess it is watch this space, but at least people are looking for solutions.

I probably have said enough on what are my views, but I hope that at some stage a government might actually consider how we may obtain food security for this increasing population while looking at some sort of self-sufficiency where possible. We cannot grow everything, but we do have a thriving livestock industry which we as vets do our best to support and make more productive while trying to maintain and improve levels of welfare on farm. We can produce to everyone's tastes of nutrition with some support and direction. And farmers can do that while also being guardians of the countryside, supporting wildlife, fauna and flora so that future generations can enjoy as much the countryside that I have grown up in and enjoyed.

A vision for the future, or just a hopeless wish? With some thought and using the natural resources available properly I am sure that we have a sustainable future, even as our population increases.

Once again, my views and now time to move on to something else!

SMALLHOLDERS:

I F MOST OF my work during my career had been working on sizeable livestock farms, then there was another part of the job which perhaps added some light relief from the intensity of working on large units. That was where the role of the smallholder came into our lives as large animal vets.

While on a stall at Minsterley Show in the summer of 2022 selling my first book, *"The Quiet Vet"* I was approached by a lady from a stall opposite us as to whether I would consider doing a talk to the local small holders' group, which attracted a membership from throughout the county. The WI had also approached me, and I was only too happy to agree to giving this talk if I was available. No timeline was given, but I did have a couple of commitments already in my diary. If we could find a mutually agreeable day then I would do so. It was eventually arranged for the beginning of October. I wondered how many of these people I would know from my working life, I would soon find out.

I wondered what they wanted me to talk about, first my experiences in Africa were mentioned as a topic but they settled on me talking about small holders and my veterinary career.

That required a bit more thought, I could have talked about Africa the whole evening without preparing anything, but now, not my specialist subject, which was a different matter. It got me thinking as to how even the definition of a small holder had changed from my early years as a child to the modern day. I was brought up on a dairy farm and in those days, we were classed as a smallholding. Dad may have started with only half a dozen cows and a few pigs and hens on his hundred- and thirty-acre farm, but we were definitely classed as a small holding, being one of the

County Council (Berkshire) smallholdings. Interestingly in some of the nearby villages of what was then a far more rural scene with no new housing estates popping up everywhere, there would be a large village green. This was often communal land, and surrounding the green there would be several of these small holdings owned by the council, a farmyard down a short stone farm track with the fields stretching out behind them. These were the smallholdings I grew up with and even when dad had over a hundred cows and numerous followers, youngstock, we were still classed as a smallholding. There was a wonderful tranquillity about them as old and traditional trees grew up in the hedgerows, gentle streams meandering through the fields with sticklebacks, bullheads, frogs, and tadpoles all at home in this English landscape.

Even when I qualified and went to work in Devon, then there were still a lot of these small family farms rented out by the council, with dairy herds of forty, fifty or sixty cows, or a few beef animals. These were still classed as smallholdings.

But I guess over time, a lot of these were sold by the council to the occupiers. Certainly, with dad's farm, there was no right of tenancy to the next generation. I had often thought of following on in dad's footsteps, as did my brothers but with no right of succession it was never going to be a feasible option. Many of the farms were bought by their occupiers and I guess when that happened, we never then thought of them as smallholdings. There maybe one or two remain but slowly but surely, they are disappearing, the days of the small holder tenant passing into history.

So, in Devon, working on smallholdings was a day-to-day occurrence, part of our bread and butter of a daily routine, going from one to another to the next door.

But that has changed now and our modern smallholder is more likely someone who has fancied the "good life" and bought a house with a few acres so that they can create a little hobby for themselves by having a few animals of their own, again whether it be a few cattle, a house cow, a few sheep, cade lambs, a few pet pigs, chickens, even alpacas and bees.

The other extreme was when I went to Kenya with *Send a Cow* to help teach their staff more about livestock farming, health, and welfare. These representatives of the charity would then go out into the local districts to reach small holders from the countries they originated from, passing on the information we had given them so that it would hopefully improve their farming, their basic nutrition and their economies so that they as a family, a community could flourish. The more and more people seeing this in their neighbourhood would hopefully follow suit. Our, the charity's aim is to take more people out of poverty, to encourage a better education, female empowerment, everything towards a better future. So here we are talking about a completely different type of small holding that may be an acre or two but may just be a small vegetable patch which will with good management and crop rotation provide food throughout the year. War rages in some of these parts so there is an unheard-of refugee crisis, but working with these small groups it is at least giving these new smallholders a beginning and a hope for the future. As the word spreads, more people want to be involved, hence the new name *Ripple Effect* to show how the work of the charity is changing from providing a goat or a cow to individual smallholders once they have shown they are willing to participate in this work, to try to improve as many people's lives as possible in one way or another, improving their agriculture.

But back to the smallholders of this country and especially in Shropshire they made a significant part of our work once we get outside of our routine visits and Tuberculin testing. A group of people with very enquiring minds who have started their own enterprises for numerous reasons, but none to make a living out of it. The wish to have a few animals of their own, a few animals for the children to look after. Visions of *"The Good Life"* from television for owners to try and be self-sufficient in some of their food supply, buying a little land with their property and having sheep to "mow the lawn", keep in shape for them. There has been no end of reasons why people have wanted their own little farm in "the back garden".

It has not been uncommon for some of these people to tell me they have started these little enterprises for wellbeing reasons. It was not that long ago that I had to visit a premises where the wife had four chickens at the end of her garden living in the most luxurious hen house I have ever seen. She wanted them because, working in a high-powered hi-tech job, she found it a retreat and very relaxing just to sit and watch them go about their daily routine. The eggs were a bonus, the therapeutic effect was the reward.

Our job was to help these willing farmers to look after and get the most out of their stock while keeping them happy and healthy. No end of them would come to our lambing courses even if they only had half a dozen ewes to lamb, they wanted to learn to be able to do it themselves, something way out of their comfort zone, rather than having to call the vet out every time.

How to use medicines, when and why and how to administer! Health programs even for the small flocks or herds and it is encouraging how many start the modern ideas such as on worming their animals, doing faecal worm egg counts to see if they need worming rather than just the regular routine dosing as done in the old days whether needed or not. A great benefit in reducing drug resistance and a big cost saver if it wasn't needed in the first place. And from my experience, one meets so many interesting people through these small holdings, people from far different ways of life but now with a few livestock of their own to keep them relaxed. Scientists, people helping to develop and trial new medicines, computer boffins, teachers, doctors, I have met people working on HS2, people helping to build nuclear reactors, environment agency workers helping to control flooding, many, many more. They have helped me to broaden my knowledge in the country I live in and given me an insight into another world that I knew very little about.

It is good that people from diverse backgrounds have found peace and tranquillity in their own farms, however big or small they may be. It does throw up one or two challenges along the way for us as vets visiting them. It maybe that what they see as an emergency late at night or over the weekend may not seem like an emergency to us as vets, but invariably we have gone out and visited them with whatever problems they may have, major or minor. But then, if they are working as well then the only time that they see their animals is outside their working hours including weekends. These times are also outside are normal working hours, but we see them anyway and this is where our role in education becomes important in teaching the owners what is important, what is not, what they can treat themselves and how, what they need to call us out for as emergencies.

But I guess the greatest challenge for us as vets is handling animals because in a lot of cases this new breed of farmer has no experience of this side of their newfound hobby and have no facilities either. Some of these places will be old farms with antiquated buildings. In those past times we would catch animals, wedge them behind gates or hurdles, or if one were available, take a student with us who was seeing practice. We must be aware of Health and Safety regulations now and so cannot approach these visits with the same gung-ho attitudes of the past. But for this new breed of clients, and they may only have a few animals then the expense of something like a cattle crush is prohibitive for the number of times it will be used. Again, education becomes important, even basic skills like how to use a halter.

It is a few years ago now, but I had to visit one client to do their Tuberculin Test. They had two Highland cattle, a beautiful breed but not always the easiest to handle. Firstly, because if they see you, they like to disappear in the opposite direction, and secondly that when adult they do have very long horns and are none too fussy what they do with them. When dealing with them, one has to be very aware where the ends of their horns are, and where you are in relation to them, especially your eyes.

This particular place, when I arrived, I was told that they had taken the trouble to build a coral and a race to catch them in with a head locking yoke at the end of the race. This should be great and straightforward, if I could just help them get the two cattle into the race. That would be no problem, only too pleased to help, although I did have it in the back of my mind a slight recollection of vets coming here in the past to do the test and the talk of tranquiliser guns! We set off across the field and when the cattle saw us, they too set off, in the opposite direction. I was shown the race from a distance and the coral and said if we could just run the cattle along the side of the fence towards the coral then we could shut the gate behind them then try and get them I not the race to test them.

A clever idea which was working well until they decided having followed the fence for a little distance, that it would be better for them if they went through the fence, not along it. Not so good, we then had to get them out of the next-door field back to where they had come from and repair the fence before trying again. It took a little time; they were certainly more agile on their feet than the four of us trying to direct them towards the coral. But patience is a virtue and at last we were successful in trapping them and shutting the gate behind them. Now to get them into the race and to Tb test them!

They volunteered themselves, heading towards the yolk where I was ready to catch the first one as it poked its head through. The owner told me that as he was well aware of their horns and if anyone needed to get behind them in the race, he had left an escape route halfway down so that a human could nip out between the gap in the race fence if necessary. It was a pity he had not thought to measure it because as the cattle went down the race, they too examined this gap....and found that they too could get through it. There was me waiting at the end, but now sadly no cattle to capture. We were back to chasing them around the field and sometime later did manage to get them back into the coral.

The office by now must have been wondering what had happened to me.

We blocked the route off, but having been that way once and got away, the cattle were only too happy to go down the race again only to find their route blocked. A bar behind them and at last we had them.

First one, head caught and me only too aware of those horns, I did what I had to do, let the first one go, trapped the second one and tested her. At last, after an hour a half I was done for what should have taken about ten minutes. Patience IS a virtue. I would have to be back in three days to read them, so suggested that we narrow the escape gap though saying it was a good idea, and we would try the same again.

It was with some trepidation that I arrived to read them, giving myself far more time to carry out the task. Luckily, the owner had managed to lure the cattle into the coral with a little food and shut the gate behind them. They were already trapped when I arrived and although they did not seem too thrilled to see me again, we were soon done and they soon admiring my departure from the other end of the field.

A mental note to myself to make sure I was away the next time it was due!

But the mention of Highland cattle takes me to a very salient point as to the value of these smallholders. We have many native breeds of sheep, pigs, and cattle but over recent years we have imported many new breeds with specific genetic traits that are deemed to be of benefit to modern production methods. With that, some of our native breeds have become exceedingly rare but it is the small holder who is having a massive part in keeping these breeds going.

I talked about pigs in *The Quiet Vet* enough, but it is nice to see such as the Wessex Saddle back, the Gloucester Old Spot, the Tamworth, all breeds of pigs that were dying out but at least we now still have a breeding population and these small holders often join breed societies soi they can keep in touch with likeminded people to ensure that these breeds persist. Who knows, one day we may want to breed back some of the traits they had into the modern pig.

I am amused that there was a craze, perhaps not so much

now that everybody wanted a Kuhn Kuhn because they were seen as mini pigs and so sweet and cuddly, especially as piglets. Some even had them as house pigs, but of course everything grows and they may not reach the size of traditional breeds of pigs, but much to the disappointment of some of their owners, they do get large. I have this wonderful picture of sitting on the settee with a two-hundred-pound pig next to you watching television, and while you want to watch Pointless or Flog It, the pig wants the controls to turn over to Peppa Pig or from way in the past, Pinky and Perky.

In mentioning the Highland cow before, others have had Gloucester Longhorns, British Whites, Dexters, and those that disappear into the distance even quicker, Belted Galloways. We see the occasional Sussex and ruby Red Devon's, all of them it is nice to think the breeds will carry on into the future.

And the same with sheep breeds. As befits the county, those that have a few Shropshires, Teeswaters, and certainly while I have worked in Shropshire, we had a few keeping the Ryeland in existence and blossoming. The Kerry, another distinctive local breed and one I had not seen much of since I was a student, and one breed that I am pleased to see again is the Hampshire, a very distinctive breed to me.

It is lovely that this small band of new farmers is making such an impact on the future of many of our rare breeds and may it long continue.

I am not an expert on poultry, but we see the same here, no end of different and unusual breeds that I have encountered especially on my Avian Flu duties.

I could think of one or two of this band of people who may have seemed a pain in the backside at times through my career but on the whole it has been a pleasure to get to know, to help and to educate these people in animal husbandry and has been a relaxing interlude away from the intensity of a lot of modern farming.

It was certainly an enjoyable evening talking to this band of people when I was asked to. And it was interesting picking up on a point that we had raised when working in Africa, and that was on the subject of co-operation and co-operatives. For these small holders, individual medicines and vaccines can be expensive on a per capita basis, making it uneconomical to use them. Pieces of equipment that may only be used once or twice in a year, again making them expensive purchases for any in dividual unit. When in Africa we often heard how these small farmers had lost goats with enterotoxaemia, and for them one goat has an appreciable part on their food supply. The loss would cause severe hardship yet there is a very effective vaccine. But it doesn't come in small units, to vaccinate a couple of animals you would have to buy enough to do twenty-five because that is how it is supplied. That makes it too expensive for an individual and we suggested that a number of them should purchase the vaccine between them, then they could all vaccinate their animals on the same day and keep the costs down. Some smallholders in this country do this, and also as a group purchase bit of equipment that they can share, again reducing costs and it became apparent talking to this group that this is what they do.

Similarly, when in Africa we discussed co-operatives as a way of selling their produce as well as group buying. There were so many advantages of working together that they could take advantage of with just a little organisation. It was more than apparent in this local group in Shropshire that they were already doing this, though not selling as a co-operative as each individual had their own reasons and their own needs from what they wanted to get out of their enterprises.

The smallholder has changed a lot from my early days but still has a significant role to play in our working lives as farm vets. Likewise, those small units at schools, at agricultural colleges, in town farms teaching the public more about the livestock they have heard of but probably never handled, the role that handling animals can have with special needs children. It all emphasises the important part that livestock can have in our lives, everybody's lives, and that we as vets have an important role in educating and improving the health and welfare of all who are involved.

If there is one regret for me in all this, I wish I knew more about bee keeping. More a specialist subject but fascinating in what I have found out about these industrious little creatures so important to pollination and all those cycles of nature. But then, a good friend has established three hives over the past year in Wales and it has been fascinating watching and helping her in her new hobby. Perhaps with a little trepidation the first time she took me to the hives hoping the bees wouldn't be too angry to see us, but they soon got used to us. Hopefully, I will gain some knowledge there. And some HONEY!

TRAGEDY:

There have been times in my career where there has been a significant loss of life on the farm, of farm stock and that has produced a significant impact of the farmer, not only for the sudden loss of his livelihood but also, and especially from the emotional attachment he or she has for their stock. I have described the impact of the epidemics that I have worked in in "The Quiet Vet". I talk of the Foot and Mouth epidemic of 2001 but have also been involved in Avian Influenza outbreaks where there has been a mass culling at infected premises. Those incidents have been heart-breaking for me as well as the livestock owner, I started in this job to save and treat animals, not to be involved in their mass slaughter. But those are the national policies involved in Notifiable Diseases in this country and you must accept that this is policy when such outbreaks take place.

But occasionally one comes across a serious disease incident, not a national incident, where through bad luck or neglect of others, a serious outcome can be produced which affects the farmer and the wellbeing of his livestock. In referring to this, I guess I am talking about toxicological incidents, poisonings. In times of little rain and drought, forage, grazing can become short and grazing livestock in their search for food will start foraging in areas that they would generally leave alone. Of course, they get supplementary feed, but by their nature they are grazers and so will start foraging around the edges of fields, through hedgerows, in fact they will look anywhere for something green. The list of plants that are poisonous is a lot longer than my long arms, but in the absence of anything else they will be eaten. Ragwort would be an example, though it affects different species differently from acute disease to causing essentially chronic liver failure. But there are others, Deadly Nightshade, Rhododendron, Hemlock, and plenty more containing well-known poisons, many which would have cropped up in the history of human crime. But of course, they grow naturally and are sometimes eaten, but in most cases causing just isolated deaths.

Toxicology is a subject in itself, and in my years, I would have tried to treat many cases of individual poisonings. Having said that, it was not uncommon for the presenting symptom to be sudden death.

There have been other times when the cause of poisoning has been accidental, feeding too much copper in the diet would be an example, especially in sheep where some breeds are more susceptible to its affects than others (were we not taught as students that if supplementing the mineral, make sure it is only given in one form). In trying to treat a deficiency, sometimes the opposite has been created and you are suddenly looking for the antidote, something that will bind up the excess mineral in the blood stream.

Many areas in our country are deficient in different minerals, plus you must take into account how other minerals can impact on the absorption of the deficiency you are trying to treat. This farm was noted for having mineral problems, notably copper deficiency plus some of the factors which inhibit copper absorption into the body, complex interactions between different elements, especially notorious on peaty soils. Nothing is easy!

It was one Good Friday, ten or twelve years ago; I was on call the Thursday night but not over the Easter weekend. Just before I was about to finish my duty and hand over to one of the other vets for the Bank Holiday, I received a phone call from one of our farmers, reporting he had a cow that was acting in a strange way, wild, manic, staggering. Could someone come out?

I should give some background to the farm and what it was trying to achieve. John had farmed there for a number of years, with a pedigree beef suckler herd. His aim was to produce high quality pedigree bulls to sell on as sires to especially dairy herds, high quality breeding heifers to sell onto other likewise pedigree breeders. So, we were looking at high quality and valuable animals on his farm. He ran a herd of about fifty cows, a couple of breeding bulls he used on his cows and heifers, plus their progeny which would be sold when reaching breeding age. In total there would be about one hundred and ten cattle on the farm at any given time, with calving starting in late February and going on into the summer.

My time on call that weekend had ended so I immediately passed the call on to the next vet, and from what the farmer described, it sounded like a case of Grass Staggers, Magnesium deficiency. The cow was housed though it is more commonly a disease of young spring grass, especially if a lot of Potash has been applied, but is not uncommon in beef suckler herds in late winter.

What the attending vet found when he arrived on the farm, a good forty-minute drive from our base was a horror show. Not only was this cow showing severe nervous signs, but it was obvious that there were others starting to show similar signs. An unsteadiness in their gait, was their vision quite as good as it should be, this was looking like a herd problem just affecting the adult cattle in one yard.

If that was the case, what had to be the common denominator with them, it had to be food or water, a deficiency or a poisoning. It was quickly decided the best course of action was to get the cattle out of the shed and away from their food source onto a clean pasture, ungrazed now since the previous autumn. The cow, which was showing signs of illness, on the basis that common things occur commonly, and her symptoms largely fitted those of Grass Staggers, was treated accordingly. In her volatile state, treatment was difficult but at last was accomplished. She was turned out with the others onto pasture. She went berserk, crashing around uncontrollably before charging through a barb wire fence and then dropping down dead. There was nothing more that could be done for her, but what about the rest of the cows. Observing them over the course of a period it became increasingly clear that their condition was deteriorating as well. Some of them seemed to be getting manic as well, more unsteady on their feet, walking around as if they did not know where they were going, losing their co-ordination and seemingly blind. These cows were heavily in calf, what was in front of the vet and John looked very serious, the whole breeding herd could be affected. Other differential diagnoses needed to be considered and Lead poisoning looked like a strong possibility. But there had to be a source, and as only the cattle in this one shed were affected, then the most likely source had to be the food, the baled silage they had in front of them in their yard.

Lead poisoning used to be a quite common occurrence especially in youngstock, calves, where they were kept in buildings and where those buildings were painted with lead paint, especially the woodwork, the doors, and frames. Calves would lick these, absorbing the mineral through their but and into their bodies. Other sources have been found to be from piping and old batteries that have inadvertently been chopped up in silaging or hay making, getting into the cattle's' food supply. There have been other reported cases and I have seen a couple where an animals water source has been a stream, and the spring that supplies it has risen or has run through an old lead mining area, producing low levels of the mineral which slowly over time build up in the animals body.

Cattle were showing clinical signs at an alarming rate, not all of these adult cattle but a sufficient number to suggest that we were dealing with a serious incident and that more help was needed. A phone call was made and the vet on second call was summoned to lend a hand with this impending disaster.

If it were lead poisoning, and that seemed the likely scenario, then treatment was needed on a herd basis, all the cattle in that shed. There is a specific antidote to lead poisoning, a drug called Calcium Versenate using its short name, a drug that when injected into the blood stream will chelate the lead, bind it to it, taking it out of the blood stream and removing its toxicity. In my early days in Devon where calves licking lead paint off doors was not

131

that uncommon, we always carried plenty on the shelf in our drugs storeroom. Since then, it has been very infrequent that I have seen a bottle, let alone had to use it. Cases of lead poisoning have become less common over time as there have been changes in paint manufacturing and calf house design. I did still have a couple of bottles in my car, but they were way out of date, I had never thrown them away (discarded them through the right channels) just in case one day I may see another case of lead.

It was of course a Bank Holiday weekend and nowhere would be open to try and get a couple of bottles, let alone enough to treat this number of cows. Was there an alternative, there is one antibiotic which will bind to lead, but whether it would bind enough only trying it would tell. A process of getting the cows back in off pasture and injecting them all intravenously was initiated; the second vet having brought vast supplies over with him from base. This was not the easiest task, not only were the cattle reluctant to come back in off grass but for those showing symptoms, handling was the last thing they appreciated, let alone having to inject large quantities of the drug into their vein, this requiring a lot of restraint.

Of course, again being a Bank Holiday, the other problem was getting a definitive diagnosis either by post-mortem of the dead cow or by biochemical analysis which would not be quick even on a normal day. That would have to wait until the Tuesday at the earliest, treatment would have to be based on clinical signs alone for the time being. But it was thought pretty definitely that lead was the culprit.

The laborious task of injecting all the cows was eventually completed, only time would tell now whether it would work or not. Veterinary assistance had gone as far as it could for that day, all one could do was to keep in touch as to the cows' progress and to revisit the following day to reassess the situation.

This left John alone on his farm with his wife and this developing situation going on in front of him. Overnight would see more fatalities. This is one of those frustrating cases of being a vet where you feel so helpless, you are relying on a second-best drug that may or not work. Even ringing around other local practices to see if they had any Calcium Versenate on the off chance that they may have some, this drew an unsuccessful outcome, they all were in the same position of not having the drug, not even knowing if it was still available.

As the Bank Holiday weekend progressed, the situation only got worse more cows showing symptoms, more cows dying. And in that another situation was developing, these were big adult cows, and the number of deaths was increasing drastically. Disposing of the bodies is carried out by a firm just over the border in Wales. But the numbers that were dying meant that several journeys would be necessary just because of the weight of animal. The other problem was that with the possibility of these carcases being contaminated with lead (and samples were taken for laboratory analysis when the labs re-opened), then incineration was the only option of disposal.

If the thought of losing all these valuable cattle was not enough, the sight of increasing numbers of bodies in the yard added to the distress of John and his family.

My involvement started after the Bank Holiday. I had been told what had happened over the weekend, but I would be going out to see another couple of cows, one slightly unsteady on her feet, the other now recumbent and had been for over twenty-four hours. Yes, I did have my out-of-date drug in the car, was it still effective and how would I decide which of the two was the most deserving case which would have the better chance of a positive outcome. I decided to split bit between them, the recumbent cow getting the larger share of it.

Did it make a difference, the honest answer was no. One cow died the next day, the other, the recumbent cow we shot some days later, she did not deteriorate but then neither did she show any signs of improvement. In the end the kindest thing was to put her out of her misery.

In the end John lost twenty cows, half of his breeding herd

and of course half of that year's crop of calves. Lead was found in ruminal contents on post-mortem, fragments of a lead battery. Lead was also detected on blood analysis. The tentative diagnosis was correct, but the alternative treatment ultimately proved to be unsuccessful.

Belatedly we did manage to get hold of twenty bottles of Calcium Versenate, but it was too late, and I think in time they were disposed of as they sat on the shelf in pharmacy until their expiry date was well passed.

The animal cost I have described, massive. The human cost to John and his mental state was also massive with him having to seek medical help, he was prescribed tranquillisers to help him try and overcome the emotional side of such a disaster on his farm.

As with all these things, the legal profession gets involved. Who was to blame? It had transpired that an electric fence powered by a lead battery had been removed from a field where horses had grazed, but inadvertently the battery had been left there. The grass grew, covered the battery, and the field of grass was then mowed so it could be made into silage and baled up into plastic wrapped silage bales. Modern machinery is so powerful it will mangle such things into tiny pieces. John bought the baled silage, and unwittingly fed this contaminated food stuff to his cattle. It may only have been one bale but that was sufficient to affect and kill so many of his pedigree herd.

The silage contractors accepted liability; they supplied the bales. If only life were that simple. John had twenty-five bales of the stuff left over, would he risk feeding this to the remainder of his herd. No way! The insurance company wanted him to open every bale and search for lead, like looking for a needle in a haystack and as soon as the bales were opened to the air, they would spoil anyway.

There is a public health scenario that any livestock that has blood lead levels over a certain measurement, they or any of their produce can never enter the food chain for fear of the same happening to humans. This applied to a couple of the surviving stock from that yard.

The loss of income from selling pedigree animals for breeding, twenty less calves which would be sold as breeding heifers or stock bulls the following year, which had to be a consideration.

I and my colleagues ended up drafting many reports of the disease incident, clinical opinions, and outcomes. Questions passed backwards and forwards from the legal profession to us, and it forever seemed as if they were trying to wriggle out of their obligations while still charging astronomical fees for their services. This went on for months and months and months, and eventually it was decided that the case would go to court. Dates were set, cancelled, and reset. In the end a settlement was reached out of court purely because John wanted a conclusion to it all. The mental stress, the mental anguish was becoming too much for him, he just wanted an end to it all.

The cost to him, both financially and emotionally were immense. And all just because someone had inadvertently left an electric fence battery in a field and forgotten about it!

Fortunately, cases like this are rare but they do happen. More usually than not, it is not deliberate, but it does happen. The outcome was tragic in this case and if nothing else, I hope it underlines the care that we as humans must take to ensure incidents like this can be avoided. They should not happen.

HIGH NOON:

A s a vet, our job is to save animals lives, to treat them in sickness, to look after their welfare, maintain their health and in the case of farm livestock, working with the farmer, trying to maximise their productivity in whatever system they are kept in. But of course, not every case can be successful despite our best efforts, animals die and for welfare reasons, if an animal is suffering then we do have to euthanase both beloved pets and productive farm livestock. One thing we are lucky with, unlike in the medical profession is that we do have the right to euthanase patients, to terminate life if that sis the best option but it can still be a very emotional occasion.

With small animals where it is the administration of a barbiturate overdose administered into a vein and the animal quietly goes to sleep never to wake, it is a peaceful way to go for the animal, minimum distress hopefully, quick, and not traumatic. But for the owner it can still be distressing, the emotional attachments that they have formed with their pet over years can be heart wrenching and in my small animal days there will have been many occasions where the emotional grief of the owner has been hard to deal with. Grown men and women crying over their loss, and in my time, I would have put to sleep dogs and cats of family and close friends, as well as those belonging to clients. It has always been a tough time to cope with, especially when your best mates are in tears.

But at least going to sleep in the arms of someone the animal trusts is a peaceful way to go. There are now plenty of pet crematoriums and memorial gardens where they can be remembered.

In farm and large animal work it is not so straight forward, firstly because of the size of the animal and secondly with what to do with the body. If injected with barbiturates one must administer large volumes and then the body would have to be incinerated because of those drugs in the body. The alternative is the use of a bullet, whether using a captive bolt to stun the animal first or the use of a free bullet.

Was I lucky while growing up on a farm that I never saw one of dad's cows shot, did it never happen, or I just was not around if it did? I do not know but cannot recollect the necessity for this to happen on farm.

So, my first experience of seeing an animal shot was when I was seeing practice as a fourth-year student at an equine practice in Lambourn. One spring Saturday morning an old horse was brought into the practice, he had come to the end of his days and the decision had already been made that this would be his last day. He was brought out of his horse trailer and being reassured by the excellent horse handlers they had at the practice, he was quietly led out into the middle of a paddock, suffering with his arthritis. With the handler standing to one side but continually reassuring the horse the vet quietly approached. I observed from a distance, in front of the horse as he ate his last few mouthfuls of grass. Not quite noon, but not far off it, the gun was raised, the end of the barrel placed on his forehead and the trigger squeezed. The sound of a gunshot and it was all over. But what surprised me, even horrified me was the sudden collapse of this once magnificent animal as his legs gave way under him and he fell in a heap onto the ground. He was dead but it seemed such an instantaneous, such a dramatic ending. The finality of a life of a faithful nag, that image stuck in my mind for many years.

I suppose since then that I have always had a hate of firearms and a reluctance to have to use one myself. But of course, we qualify and then that task, euthanasia becomes a part of our job, a necessity that we have to perform from time to time, especially in small animal practice (but not with a gun). I cannot remember the first time that I would have had to put to sleep a dog or cat, but the worry being a new graduate was always that you could find the vein easily (sometimes not easy in an animal with reduced blood pressure or terminally ill) so that a smooth ending to life could happen.

The worry of that first farm or large animal was far more daunting. In *"The Quiet Vet"* I have described having to attend a very valuable three-day event horse, called out by the police as it had been involved in a traffic accident and looked like it had a broken leg. My first experience would not only be of this valuable animal but also observed by the boys in blue, enough to make anyone more than a bit nervous. The horse had actually dislocated its fetlock and I managed to manipulate it back into place, strap it up and it lived to continue its career as an eventer. I had been saved the ordeal and was truly thankful.

We were then in Devon a large farm practice and there were other avenues of disposing of these casualties, slaughter men in the vicinity or the local hunt would come out and euthanase livestock for the farming community.

So, my next experience would be a horse again, but this time a horse with severe colic which it was not going to recover from, caused by a twisted gut. The horse was owned by a young lady, not a girlfriend but more than an acquaintance which did not make the decision any easier. Why did there always seem to be some sort of emotional attachment in these cases?

The practice had a Colt 45 which we used as a humane killer, a free bullet into the forehead at zero range, and with the horse in distress and on the ground it was an easy but unenjoyable task to dispatch him from this world, to relieve his suffering from something he wasn't going to recover from.

The task was done, all I had to do now was to comfort a thankful but upset owner. I placed the gun on top of my car while I offered comfort, at last in what had been an emotional experience for all involved, managed to make my leave, getting in my car, and driving off.

How long did it take for me to realise that the gun was not in the car, I had left it on the roof and had gone. More worry, it had to have fallen off and I would have to stop and walk back searching for the weapon. I would then be seen wandering along this main road back to the car carrying a gun. How good would that look, especially with the police station only another mile down the road.

I stopped and got out of the car, and to my surprise, and I do not know how, the gun was still where I had left it. I placed it back into the car and beat a hasty retreat to the office to replace it back in the safe from where I had got it from.

A Colt 45 sounds impressive and although I am no expert, it was a nice gun to use, but thankfully for me it was a one off, I never had to use it again in my time in Devon.

I moved on to Gloucestershire and to a mixed practice once again, and if there can be some emotion attached to the job, I do not think you would count it as memorable, but one evening surgery I had fourteen clients booked in with appointments. I did not know what they were coming for, but at the end of two hours I had seen seven dogs with bad ears and had euthanised seven digs for a variety of reasons required by their owners. Not an evening of fulfilment for the vet but that is what the paying public wanted, and you can only go so far in persuading whether it should be done or not.

I was supposed to being playing cricket that evening for a local side, my friend picked me up outside the surgery, me being a few minutes late and giving my explanation he was horrified though in later years it became a standing joke with him.

He took me down to the local golf club one Sunday, I had just started playing, and introduced me to the club captain, a man of importance with his opening line of his introduction of me being, "This is Rod Wood, I expect he has probably put your dog down"!

I had and if the ground could leap up and swallow me there and then!

At a future date at the golf club, he introduced me to another dignitary of the club with a slightly different line, "This is Rod

Wood, I expect he has put your cat down."

I had; this golf club was starting to be a real embarrassment to me. At least no-one mentioned birdies, eagles and albatrosses. I may have got into trouble with the RSPB!

But we were a mixed practice in the Forest of Dean and so would have to see all sorts of animals. Yes, the few small animals as described but essentially, I was a farm vet who may have to see a dog or cat out of hours. We did not do a lot of horse work, there was a big equine practice down the road, but we did see some horses and ponies, but nothing that was woo valuable. And that of course meant that we would have to see the odd disaster, a broken leg, a bad colic. That in turn would mean that the need for euthanasia on welfare grounds would arise again.

Our firearm in this practice I had not seen the likes of before but I suppose when you strip a gun down to its basics then it is only a tube of metal, somewhere to put a bullet and something, a pin, that will hit the bullet at force to cause an explosion that causes the release of the harmful shot.

I was called out to a pony in a nearby village that may have broken its leg. I was advised to take the gun with me and retrieved this thick cloth bag from the gun safe. I thought it best to familiarise myself with this weapon before arriving on the scene. Two metal tubes that screwed together, the barrel, one of which on the end had a pin protected by a metal loop that covered it but was retractable. A place to put the bullet within this, but how did you fire the "gun". There was a small wooden block in the bag also and what one had to do was to hit the pin with this wooden block to fire the gun. The other end was a plate with a hole in (the barrel) which one rested against the forehead of the doomed animal.

I went out to see the pony and sadly she did have a broken foreleg and would have to be euthanised. The owner was expecting this, but probably not with the contraption I got out of the bag and started assembling. I felt a little awkward but a gun is a gun, and so getting the owner to stand to the side and in front of the pony I placed this thing on the pony's head and just hoped that it would not react as it saw this bit of wood coming towards it, and that the force of my tap would be sufficient to fire the damn thing.

In fairness, it did the job it was intended for, and the poor pony was put out of its misery, to which the owner was very grateful. That hid my awkwardness in having to use this weapon.

My only other occasion was having to euthanase a goat with it. This beast was far less inclined to keep its head still while I tried to do my duty, made more difficult by the fact that the owner did not want to be present. I did manage in the end, a swift tap, bang, and hopefully job done. But here I did wonder if the "gun" was too powerful for the condemned as I am sure the bullet went straight through the head and out the other side, luckily into the ground. I had achieved what I had set out to do but it did give a warning of the dangers (if I did not know enough of them already) of using a free bullet on smaller animals.

But strangely enough again in all my time in Gloucestershire I was never called upon to have to shoot a bovine or ovine.

I would meet a similar weapon in my next practice, same basic architecture of the gun but a different piece of wood. I did have cause to use it a few times unfortunately but now with more cattle around, I would have to shoot my first cow. A daunting prospect but at least in a lot of cases in cattle, they are recumbent and the anatomical landmarks of where to shoot are very distinct. I think this gun must have been quite old, the ammunition too. I was called out one day to see a cow down in the field who had a toxic mastitis, and she was not going to recover. The farmer requested that I did the kind thing for her and if I could euthanase her. She was not going to run away so he left her to me, to dispatch her humanely.

I assembled the gun, loaded a bullet in it, placed it on her forehead and fired, a swift tap on the pin, bang, and expected all to be done. To my surprise, the cow just looked at me as if to say, "What was all that about"?

The bullet must have been a dud, it made the required noise but just left a black powder mark on the cow's forehead, an apparent blank. Thankfully the second attempt achieved the right result, but I never had any faith in this weapon again.

In time the partnership was dissolved to become just a small animal practice. We would need to get rid of the gun so it was decided that we would see if the police would accept it. I rang them to see and arrange a time to take it into them at the headquarters in town.

I arrived at the appointed time and handed the bag with the gun over, plus the remaining ammunition we had. The duty sergeant would have to give me a receipt for the gun and writing it out did have an official name for the type of weapon it was (I cannot remember its name) and then coming to the piece of wood used to hit the firing pin with.

"What shall I describe this as," he asked, "the trigger I suppose"! And that is what he recorded it as on the receipt.

I was not sorry to never see that type of weapon again in my career.

We were at a time because of various firearm incidents in the country that I would need a Firearms certificate to be able to carry and use one, along with all the necessary requirements that went with it, such as having a secure and lockable safe in the car if transporting it while driving. In my new practice ewe did cover vast distances and so especially at night and weekends it was impractical to have to go to the office every time one needed a weapon. I duly applied and was granted a certificate to use the gun the practice held, the irony I suppose being that at no time had anyone ever shown me how to use one properly, and the safety aspects I had had to work out for myself.

I did need to use it but on not many occasions but was once asked by one of my vet partners if I could take the gun upto him some twenty-five miles away urgently as he had a horse which needed shooting asap. I got the gun from the safe and in the need for haste, just had it sitting on the passenger seat of my car as I set off to this equine stables.

There was a police check point as I left the town heading

north. Help, I have a gun on my car seat! Luckily, they had no need to stop me, and I was able to proceed without having to explain this!

It was during this time that I became involved in the 2001 Foot and Mouth outbreak in the country. Vets were seconded from General practice to help out trying to control this epidemic which was sweeping the country and had arrived in Shropshire. We as a large practice in the county felt we had to support the national effort and having first sent a young American vet to help, it was then felt that we should send an experienced vet to take over for the duration of how long a vet would be needed by DEFRA. That vet was me!

But although I did this job for six weeks continuously, this would be the start of some dark days for me. If I spent the first couple of weeks going around the county where needed inspecting holdings in any Surveillance zone that had livestock, checking to make sure there was no disease on the premises, I did eventually get sent as a welfare officer to supervise the slaughter of sheep which had been traced as a possible contact. These sheep that had been sold through a Cumbrian market early in the outbreak. Here we were talking about a couple of months after that outbreak, but sheep can remain symptomless with this disease. Government policy was that all these should be slaughtered so on a sunny April morning I was sent, along with a slaughter crew, to dispatch over three thousand sheep, most of them lambs. A captive bolt was the chosen method of slaughter, a gun firing a metal pin into the brain of the condemned animal, dispatching it quickly if fired in the right place. My job was to check all this was done humanely, without causing all the animals' undue distress and to check that when shot, all these animals were dead.

It was a sole destroying and tiring job as the pile of carcases grew bigger and bigger. Was this what I had trained to do? At the time it didn't seem like it and the effects it had on my mental health have already been described previously.

But we had a job to do and had to get on and do it. How many sheep would I see over the coming days to suffer the same fate, but I did my job, just got on with it though questioning the need for it. Some of these sheep with suspect lesions did seem more traumatic to me that those caused by the disease. But I guess what did affect me the most was the use of captive bolts. I know we had a large number of animals to deal with and it is not the most stimulating of jobs but with the numbers the slaughtermen were having to deal with in a day, there were too many that needed to be shot a second time. The pressure and monotony on these men was immense and to be honest, there was no other method that we could deal with this number, but on more than one occasion we did have to stop and me ask if we could take a little more care, be a little more precise in what we were doing. The welfare of these animals was paramount, even if they were about to meet their end.

I guess I have never really had faith in captive bolts since then.

But a few days later, again as a welfare vet, I was asked to supervise the slaughter of a large dairy herd which was in the protection zone. With such an infectious disease, any livestock in a three-mile radius would have a compulsory slaughter order placed upon them and it would occur as soon as possible after an infected premises was identified to try and reduce any possible further spread.

It was a Sunday morning, the sun was shining, and we had a job to do, the next-door farm was a positive case and this was the consequence. There was a debate as to whether cattle should be slaughtered individually through the farm handling system, then the bodies carted away before the next cow would meet the same fate. But we had experienced slaughtermen here, expert riflemen and we decided that it would be quicker and cause less distress if the cows were shot where they stood. A yard could be cleared and then filled again for the process to be repeated.

I would have to say here that I was grateful for how efficiently these men did their job, expert shots who would dispatch the poor animal from a short distance, but they were good shots and would just drop to the ground as their mate standing next to them just carried on chewing her cud as if nothing had happened. It was quick, efficient and there was no suffering, my inspection of these animals was quick and easy, the necessary job had been done and there was no need for further intervention.

Over the coming weeks I would get use to this and their efficiency in what was not a pleasant task but it had to be done. There were occasions when, and we did work as an efficient team now especially after the army got involved as well, I was asked if I would like to have a go with one of the guns. I had a Firearms certificate and so would be allowed to use one of these rifles. Every time I was asked, I graciously declined. I had to be there to supervise this slaughter, but I could not do it myself. These men were trained, well-practised but I was not. Supposing I missed or was not quite accurate enough, the animal could suffer. On top of that, I was still not completely happy in my mind that all this was necessary. That is not doubting our national policy, it was just that in some of these cases I was not absolutely sure in my mind that it was Foot and Mouth we were dealing with. There was an emotional side to this, both to the owner whose livestock livelihood was being destroyed, as well as to me and my mental health. I was classed as "dirty" because of my potential contact with the disease so couldn't go back to my practice, couldn't meet other veterinary colleagues still working in practice, nor meet any farmer friends. They certainly did not want to see me and risk the possible carriage of infection to their stock.

Dark days.

The lasting affects for me, I have never used a captive bolt since, though many of my colleagues have done. For me, I have preferred the use of a free bullet and its greater efficiency though having to be aware of the greater safety requirements involved in this method.

I can recall a couple of incidents in the past where there have been problems.

One day I was called out to see a heifer with a suspected broken leg. In those days I only took the gun when I needed to and would be fairly sure that the diagnosis given would be correct. On seeing this beautiful animal, nearly ready to calve for the first time one didn't need to be a brain surgeon to confirm that this foreleg dangling there was well and truly bust, and there was only one thing we could do. She was suffering so it was not fair on her to call the local slaughter man, she would have to be shot there and then.

Our difficulty was that of approach. Pain can do strange things to behaviour and in this heifer's pain, her temperament had changed drastically. Normally a calm animal, she now in pain had turned into a vicious animal. Despite only being on three legs she would just face us and if we approached to close, she would go for us.

What should we do? I had a revolver and needed to direct it at her forehead from close range and she was not going to let me get close. We did not have anything like a dart gun to sedate her first, but the farmer, Jim, did have his own rifle. Our plan we decided was that he would shoot her from distance, hopefully into the heart then I would approach rapidly when she had fallen and shoot her in the normal way.

The first shot she did drop but with me approaching, she did try to get to her feet. I had to retreat. The second shot, success and I was able to approach and finish the job.

On another occasion I had one night gone to visit a cow that was down. From my examination, she was never going to stand again, and it would have been wrong to let her live any longer. I would shoot her. But how long did it take me to persuade the farmer that he really did not want to stand behind her, right in my line of fire. After minutes of persuasion, I did at last get him to stand behind me well out of the danger area.

Over my final years in practice, I did have to use a gun from time to time when necessary, renewing my Firearms Certificate when necessary, always stating on the application that it was for use in protecting the welfare of livestock where humane destruction was necessary. I used the firearm of another vet, my name being added to the use of that weapon, but through that time I was never allowed access to his other firearms. As it should be.

Retirement came and I would have to admit that I was glad to hand the gun back to its rightful owner, I would never have to use it again.

And I will gladly surrender my Firearms certificate. I have always felt uncomfortable with a gun and will happily give up the responsibility of having one in my possession. Its use has been necessary at times in my career but not something I shall miss.

High Noon!

TB TESTING:

I GUESS THAT takes me onto the other guns I have used through my career, Tb testing guns, or syringes, whichever one wants to call them. Tuberculin testing has been mentioned several times throughout my tale, and somewhere I do have to write about it as it has taken up such a large proportion of my life, of any farm vet's life. But at the present time, with differing intervals between tests depending on where abouts you are in the country, all cattle more than likely will be tested at least once in their lives.

In my last position in Shropshire, we are a Tb area and so all farms have to be tested very six months unless classed as an infected premises, have had at least one reactor in a previous test in which case they will be tested every sixty days until there have been a series of clear tests, depending on individual situations which Animal Health will decide. Ultimately, all decisions are made by them, we just perform the tests, reading and interpreting the results as to whether the cow has passed or is a reactor.

In my early days in Devon our main work outside day to day farm work was more involved with Brucellosis testing, taking blood from heifers over eighteen months old to see if they had antibodies against this infectious disease causing infertility and abortion in cattle, but also being a disease that can affect humans, Undulant Fever. This we would have to do annually back in those days, Tb testing on adult cows and calves which had not been out to grass every two years. How things have changed.

The Foot and Mouth outbreak in 2001 meant vast areas in the country had their cattle population reduced from the compulsory slaughter policy, and to restock these farms, cattle were bought in from elsewhere in the country and some of those areas would be found out to be infected areas for Tb. Rapidly, the disease was spread to areas that did not previously have a problem. They did now. Areas such as the one I had worked in Devon had become problem areas and it has taken a lot of time and effort to reduce the incidence of disease. Gloucestershire where I had worked was known to be a problem area and there had been a badger cull project back in the seventies to see if by reducing the badger population, the disease in cattle would be reduced as well. There was a defined link between badger and cattle.

Over the years this link has become an emotive subject and one cannot deny that with a far greater badger population once it became a protected species, the incidence of Tb in cattle also rose markedly. Similarly, it must be said that badgers are not the only wildlife species that have been shown to carry Tb. It was found in Gloucestershire that in one studied colony, that badgers could travel miles at night to feed, especially when the found that delicacy for them of maize, corn on the cob.

But as I have said, it is an emotive subject, and even if a badger cull has had positive effects in reducing bovine Tb in some areas, that debate will go on and it is not for me to expound theories or opinions here. All one can say is that the disease in cattle will be a problem for some time to come, testing will go on, research into better testing will go on and that one day we may see a vaccine against it. But talk of a vaccine has been going on for years, some twenty-five years ago I heard a talk where they said it was fifteen years away, ten years later it was fifteen years away. Now, who knows?

So, it has become an emotive subject throughout society, but one should also think hard about those people it affects, the farmer. Over my years in practice, how many farmers have I seen break down in tears when you have completed their test and have had to inform them that they have a reactor, the cow would have to be slaughtered. The farm will then be shut down in terms of selling other cattle unless going direct to slaughter as in the case of beef animals. The number of animals on the farm will increase until clear again and this will cause hardship both in terms of welfare, stocking density, more feed needed, more work, and the financial implications to the business with increased costs and loss of income. I, as many other vets will have done, have performed tests that when reading the results of the skin test, haven't even needed to have had cattle reach the crush to read them to see that they had got huge lumps on them and when they got to me to be read, I already knew that they had failed. They were reactors. Tests where ten, twenty, thirty, even eighty cows in one go would fail and must go, heart breaking for us vets and even more so to the farmer who has bred and reared them.

Some would not believe the results of the test, even though it was in front of their eyes, some would blame us the vets performing the test for the results, we had not done the test properly and some just had no faith in the test anyway. That made it hard on us doing the test and with that we would get complaints and abuse. It should be said that those cases were the minority, but it still did not make our job any easier. There would be many who accepted that sooner or later they would get Tb on their farm, others with the distress that it caused them, then we would have to hard job of trying to reduce the emotional upset it was causing them.

The other problem for us would be those cows that were slaughtered after failing their test only to go to the abattoir and no lesions of the disease would be found, nor could the bacteria that causes Tb be grown in the lab. There are explanations for this like it being in the very early stages of infection, but it was always hard to get a farmer to except these explanations.

It has and will remain so an emotive problem that the rural farming community will have to deal with for some time, it would be nice to think that sometime in the future we will get on top of Tb and finally eradicate it from these shores but we are still a long way from that.

But despite the days, years of monotony Tb testing, and there have been many of them, it has also provided days of amusement, jollity along with times of frustration and a test on my patience.

Some of my testing days have been described in previous chapters in this book and the last, one or two I will mention now.

An introduction to the rare breeds of Britain has been an advantage of my testing days. Those days having to deal with those breeds of our native isles with long horns has at times been challenging. Such as the Longhorn I have found to be quite docile animals, and the likes of Rob and Sam who have bred these cattle would always have a respect for them although they were on the whole co-operative in what you were trying to do to them. I found their one failing was that though they had these long horns, their spatial awareness with them was not great and if they turned their heads, they did not really appreciate where the end of their horns were. Where this mattered was that because of the length of them, it was not always easy to get them in a modern cattle crush, let alone trap their heads in the yoke to be able to carry out the skin Tb test.

I spent a wonderful autumn afternoon having to test over a hundred of these Longhorns in a parkland setting where there was a coral and a race, with a yoke of sorts at the end of it. The older cows with their long horns would make their way down the race, turning their heads from side to side to manoeuvre themselves and their horns to the end. One could risk trying to yoke them but if they barged through then they were gone, free to roam the parkland. It was easier just to keep the gate shut at the front of the race and test them with their heads unrestrained. Leaning over the railings, for me the tester, I just had to watch where the tips of the horns were, they always seemed to be at eye height. It was a peaceful afternoon in what is brilliant old English parkland, surrounded by magnificent old oak trees, treading over multiple acorns which were now falling to the ground. Wonderful, until the heavens opened, and we all got soaked. Did it worry the cattle, no, but for me trying to test them, watching out for their horns while my glasses needed windscreen wipers, rainwater penetrating my waterproofs, running down my back and also into my boots, well! And the paperwork I was trying to complete, recording the skin readings (and I was also blood testing the cattle for other diseases), despite keeping it as sheltered in the cab of the farmer's truck, it was impossible to keep dry, the longer I tested, the more and more these pages got stuck together, and the harder it became to write upon them. Of course as we finished, the sun came out again and I had to peel the sheets away from each other laying them on the back seat of my car separately, hoping when I got home I would still be able to decipher enough of what I had written to start afresh on new sheets all I had recorded.

Despite the rain, it was a lovely environment to work in.

These were placid animals, my experiences with the likes of Highlands were different and have been mentioned before. They seem quite different in this environment compared with those I have seen grazing contently in fields in Scotland with calf at foot, resting under trees or scratching themselves against fence posts or just standing admiring their surroundings. Perhaps they would have been different if I had needed to do anything to them, but I was on holiday, it wasn't my job.

I had seen Belted Galloways across the valley when my parents first moved to Exmoor and had often admired their beauty. As a vet, it was a breed I had little to do with, when in Shropshire, I had one smallholder who had a few of these cattle. They were his hobby and my only contact with them would be for their annual Tb test. From my limited experience, I think they would have to be the wildest breed I have come across. There may only have been half a dozen of them to test but I needed to allow myself a lot of time to do them. I think it would be true to say that we saw far more of their backsides as they disappeared over the brow of the hill again as we tried to get them into a shed to test. A breed that once you had got them in, you would not risk that trick of opening the crush gate slightly to try and get them to enter it, if they charged forward, they were gone and that view of their rear ends over the hill would reappear! They were lovely to see as a breed, not great to do anything with and for this reason, despite his love of the breed, the farmer did not keep them for very long. I think my next experience of them was on a beautifully picturesque walk in Borrowdale up in Lakeland where they stood between me and a small stone bridge I needed to cross. Four of them, and as I approached, they were quite happy to carry on chewing the cud, letting me pass without batting an eyelid. So peaceful, so calm and a prelude to what was the most amazing scenery of my walk that day.

Devon's (wild), South Devon's (not), British Whites (long horns again) and the more traditional breeds of Herefords, Angus, Jersey, Guernsey, Shorthorn and then of course came the Continentals. I must not forget those few Dexters that I have had to test, our smallest breed and even for me of no great height, one would have to get on your knees to be at a height that you could test them.

In the embryonic stages of my career, I was called once to one of our farmers in Devon to see a cow that appeared to be poisoned. In those days of traditional farming, small paddocks surrounded by hedgerows and trees, especially in times of a lack of rain, sometimes to a cow the best grazing would in their minds be in these hedgerows, and in there would often be plants that were no conducive to good health. In those Devon summers, cases of plant poisonings were not uncommon. I had it somewhere in my mind from my university days that certain of these plants, the toxins they contained could be precipitated out using tannins. Where would I get these tannins from, much to the farmer's surprise I asked him to bring me some freshly brewed tea and a lot of it. The look on his face was that why should I want a cuppa now when I should be treating his poorly cow but after explaining what I wanted it for, he went off and came back with jugs full of tea….and a cuppa for himself and me. The three of us enjoyed our afternoon tea although as we sipped ours from a mug, the cow had hers poured down her throat with a stomach tube. A few hours later the farmer rang me and informed me the cow was far better, the tea had worked, and he was very grateful.

He became a farmer I got on well with and a few weeks later I had to go back to his farm to do his Tb test on his cattle, cows, and the young calves. The easiest way of testing the cows was to put them through his Abreast parlour, few of them seen these days but back in the eighties very common especially on his size of farm where they were milking eighty to a hundred cows. In fact, it was the type of parlour I was used to from dad's farm. The cows stood on standings either side of a food dispenser, also where the milking machine apparatus was. A cow would be milked on one side of this standing while the next cow stood the other side, being prepared for milking. Depending on the size of the herd, which would determine how many of these standings there were, in this case four units so eight cows could be in the parlour at a time. By blocking one side of each standing off, we could get four cows in at a time, I could Tb test them, record what I had to and then let them out of the exit door and bring in another four. In theory, extremely easy and quite quick as the cows were used to going through the parlour, far more used to it than going through a cattle crush one at a time.

We started the test and it was going well, but in any herd of cows you have the ones that are keen to go through and they are the first to enter, then you are left at the end with the shy cows, the nervous ones, those that always seem to be a bit more flighty. We had noticed as we worked our way through the herd that the doorway was taking a little collateral damage as cows pushed through to get in the parlour. Now we were just left with a few at the end, those suspicious cows that on taking a look at the change in the parlour, and with me a stranger standing in there as well, no sooner had they entered than they changed their minds and in unison headed straight back towards the door they had just entered through. With all that weight arriving at once, as they pushed their way out into the yard again something had to give, and it did. With their combined push, the strength of the cement holding together the breeze blocks making up the front of the parlour was tested beyond what it could take. Part of the front of the parlour collapsed onto the yard, other of the bricks were just left hanging loosely on top of each other.

We now had an open plan parlour and before we could finish the test would have to tidy up what was left of the wall, protect it with gates, and when all was safe, we finished off the test on these last few reluctant cows who quite approved of the openness of the parlour now.

There was good humour about it, the farmer had expected it to happen for some time and had spoken to his landlord about it several times. Over another cuppa, we discussed it, had a laugh about it, especially as nobody had been hurt.

When I returned three days later, behold, he had a new parlour wall, strong and reinforced so the same would not happen again. The cows all passed their test, the building was now safe and through this mishap, the landlords had at last done the repairs they had promised to do for so long.

I wonder in all my years as a vet while I was testing, how many other buildings were left in not quite the same shape as when I had arrived on the farm, there were several and luckily no one or no animals were hurt on any of those occasions.

Perhaps in those days we were very gung-ho about testing and the animal handling facilities we worked with. Health and Safety now becomes a large part of any job we do, having to do a risk assessment on the facilities we have available to us. We are quite in our rights to refuse to do a test if we consider facilities unsafe and that sometimes can cause a little friction between the tester and the farmer. I have generally got on with what has been handed to me but there have been incidences where I have said that something needed to be improve the next time I was there, or if another vet came, they may refuse to work in those conditions. We have to look after ourselves and any helpers, ultimately it is our responsibility.

I may have mentioned already the injuries us vets get when testing, and occasionally we would get as a practice an email from APHA enquiring about any that may have occurred while we were carrying this work out for them. My ailments have generally not stopped me working, the bang on the head sent me home early and the aftereffects of the neck injury incurred at the same time I suffered from then, and still do. It will affect me for the rest of my life with trips to the chiropractor necessary from time to time when I find I cannot turn my head fully, not good when you are driving. The odd times that I have been trapped by a large bovine against a gate or rails when it has pushed through before its turn while I have been testing another animal, especially if I have been doing another procedure at the same time like blood testing, then I have just carried on, even if feeling a little bruised. Not so long ago in my career I was testing a beef herd, and blood testing the herd at the same time for their High Herd Health status annual test, and pregnancy testing a few as they went through as well. It was an efficient cattle handling system with a metal barrier that slid down behind the cow as she entered the crush. The next cow waited behind this barrier for her turn to come. I had tested the cow in the crush and was extracting blood from her tail vein. The cow behind was getting impatient and cleverly managed to lift the barrier up with her head, once up a little she was able together head right underneath it, lift it fully and walk forward. She wanted to be out and gone but with a cow in front of her, the best she could do was to press up as close behind her as she could. Except between the two cows was me, and as the second cow pressed more and more forward, the space I had diminished considerably. The owners were concerned for my safety but there was no obvious solution to my plight. There was no room for me to try and slide back and get out of the side gate, the second cow was persistent in her efforts to push forwards and the cow at the front was yoked in, if we let her go then she would go forward with the other cow right behind her and would take me with her as she went forward. I could fall and be trampled on or just crushed further.

Was I starting to panic abit, very probably. We, I should say the farmer tried driving the second cow backwards, but she only had one thing on her mind and that was escaping forwards. She was stubborn! I had managed to get enough blood from the cow I was testing but then had my arms down by my side. I was well and truly trapped. I am not a big person, perhaps losing a couple of pounds around the waist wouldn't hurt me and perhaps I was lucky because I was small. I do not really know how I managed it but after a couple of hair-raising minutes, with a bit of wriggling this way and that, I did manage to squeeze out through the side gate. I was lucky because for more than a few seconds I could not see a way out, and despite all the efforts of the farmer and his helper, they couldn't budge the second cow such was her determination to be out and gone.

A lucky escape, and after a couple of minutes I dusted myself down and continued, I still had a lot of cows to test before I was finished. A lucky escape indeed.

But these things happen and despite our attention to health and safety these days, some accidents, however much you try, are unavoidable. Other colleagues in their time will have had nasty leg injuries, arm injuries, kicks, an endless list and following these incidents, have been unable to work for days or weeks afterwards.

It is a repetitive job, the same actions time after time, day in and day out so repetitive stress injuries are common. Again, time off and then physio being necessary before one can contemplate a return to work.

And because of the repetition of the job, it can get very boring doing it day in and day out. I was a clinical vet as well so would have a mix of testing, my routine work and fire brigade work, dealing with any emergencies that may come in. We employed several vets whose sole job was Tb testing and for them there did seem to be a finite time that they could continue doing this same job four days a week and throughout the year before looking for other areas of employment in the veterinary profession. Three, four years seemed to be enough. A lot of these vet testers tended to be foreign vets who had come over here because of the lack of vet work in their home countries, especially Spain and Romania. They have struggled with the language to begin with, farmers also struggling to understand their tongue but when barriers have been broken down, they have in the end been popular.

Now, especially after Brexit, even their numbers have diminished and practices are allowed to employ non-vets to carry out this work, though they still need training from vets, and their work signed off by us. How long they will find they can do the job, time will tell. It is good that many of those European vets that I have known as Tb testers who have remained in this country are now finding work as clinical vets, the job they trained to do.

One advantage they do have now is the advancement in electronic technology. When I started, and for many years of my career, one had to do all the paperwork manually, a long and laborious job especially on some of the large herds we have now. Writing each ear number, breed, age, sex and their skin readings took forever. We were then able to do it all on computer with the program generating lists of cows for you, you just had to fill in the readings. Since my retirement, the tester now has a handheld cow side device which produces this list, by filling in a few of the numbers on the tag you can find the cow and only have to fill in the readings. When finished, linking this to the computer program, at the press of a button it is all loaded, filled in and one can send the report off straight away. How much easier is that than what us older vets had to deal with for most of our career.

Health and Safety, wrecking buildings and farm "furniture", doing battle with wild cattle have all added to the excitement of Tb testing over the years, even if now the chance of finding reactors in herds in the area I have worked has increased dramatically. As I have said before, it has been a case of when, not if you get Tb in your herd. This has made the task of completing all this testing more exacting as why a greater number of recruits have been needed to conduct all this work. In infected areas we are not now testing just adult cattle and any youngsters which have not been out to grass, but any bovine on the premises that is over forty-two days old. Bigger herds, more cattle to test on each farm and at more regular intervals on infected farms, I wonder just how many animals get tested in the practice I worked in every year. Thousands and thousands. As well as that, as part of the control method, pre-movement testing was introduced to try and prevent the spread of the disease. Farms not under restrictions, if they wanted to sell cattle at market or sales, they would have to have any cattle over that forty-two day old age tested before they could leave the farm. If these animals were clear, then they could be sold to another farm, and it would give some peace of mind to the purchaser that they were not buying in disease.

More cattle to test, though usually less of a strain and more relaxed as it was more than likely these cattle would pass their tests, usually being young and from an already clear farm. I think in all my time doing pre-movement tests, there were only a couple of times that I picked up either inconclusive or reactor cattle meaning that the farm would be shut down for moving cattle on. These pre-movement tests tend only to be a few cattle, a few calves so could easily be fitted in between other calls, depending on where they were relevant to other calls you were doing.

So vast number of cattle to test and to be able to do that, especially with the large herds we have now, meant very early starts. When I started as a vet all those years ago, with smaller herds and less cattle required to be tested on each farm, we invariably started a Tb test after the farmer had finished milking and had had his breakfast. Now, especially with some of these massive herds where they are milking eight hundred to a thousand cows, an early start is required which means testing the cows during milking time. The cows are milked and then that group that has just left the parlour is forwarded towards the race and cattle crush and tested straight away before heading off for her morning feed or a return to grass. When all the milking cows are done, then we go onto the youngstock to test which may mean moving all the cattle handling equipment elsewhere and setting it up (time for some breakfast while the farm staff do this) or having to go and round up youngstock out of a field, even set up the equipment in a corner of the field they are in. Very time consuming.

But again, the strain on Tb testers having to start their day early, day in, day out, is immense. I know the farm workers have to do it every morning, and although the early morning starts were tried to be divided out equally so there could be some break from it, it is something else that impacts on your life.

Early morning starts were something that never worried me that much, but then I didn't have to do the number the Tb tester vets did, and the ones that I did do were more than often for the clients that I did most of their work, so the atmosphere was more relaxed and I knew their systems. I am a poor sleeper, and I do not think there was ever one occasion where I had to be woken to go and do an early morning test. It was a real pain knowing you had to get up at three, three thirty in the morning and going to bed early to try and get some sleep only to watch the clock go round and switch the alarm off before it would go off. Frustrating, even more so if I was on call the following night, the next evening off and then the following morning an early start on that same farm again.

I had a farm where there would be over fifteen hundred cattle to test, and they started milking at five o'clock in the morning. For me to get there to start the test it would mean getting up at just after three, having a small breakfast (I knew I would get a cooked breakfast on the farm when we had finished testing the milkers) before making the thirty-five mile journey to the farm. Sometimes it was a bit disheartening to find the place in total darkness, I was the first person to be at the farm. Two of us would usually do this test together, I had the pleasure of working it with my Spanish comrades, first Pablo, then Pelayo and we managed to work a system that we could get through the cows quickly and efficiently so that when milking had finished, then we would be finished almost straight away afterwards. While the staff were swapping milking groups, I would go and test the young calves so by ten o'clock we would have done all the cows and babies at the main farm. We had a good system, and the staff were used to us, so we got on well, and even if it was monotonous, it was good humoured, we had a laugh while we were testing, even though the staff didn't enjoy seeing us every sixty days.

When we had finished there and had our breakfast, Pablo, Pelayo, which ever it was, and I would then part company each with a team of helpers to go and test the heifers which were scattered around different parts of the county either at heifer rearers or at grass keep. We wouldn't see each other again that day, sometimes we finished at the same time, other times I would be far later as my last group to test were over the border in Wales, and often on this part of the test I would have to pregnancy diagnose some of the heifers as well. We always had a café stop on the way where we would stop for a bacon or sausage bap and a coffee.

It could be a long and tiring day, even more so in earlier days when I did the test by myself so often finishing in the late afternoon or early evening. On one test I finished the last lot of heifers in late spring when they were out at grass, arriving at their field at dusk and having rounded them all up into a coral, tested them in the dark. An early start and a very late finish, which was a tiring day.

But one thing I would have to say with places like this was how well organised they were. Okay, we were testing on these big farms at regular intervals, so they were used to it and had adapted a handling system to suit all concerned, but it still required a good deal of humour and management to work it efficiently and safely.

There were other places though where another talent was required, and that was patience. If there were two things often commented about me, it was firstly how quiet I was and second, my patience was often noticed and praised. A test like the one above was long but well organised. If I did get there sometimes before anybody else did, it was not because they were late, more likely that I was early. But when you arrive at an appointed place on time and there is nobody to be found or if they are a long way from being ready, then it could be very frustrating, especially if I had a long list of other calls to do when I had finished that Tb test.

Did I ever lose my temper, I think the answer to that was a no, even if inside me there was a real sense of annoyance. It would be the last Tb test I ever did, helping the practice out after retirement, but was a good example of either inefficiency or being taken for granted. I had been given a large test to do, split over two days as there were cattle in several places. The Monday test was due to start at four in the morning, doing the cows as they came out of the parlour. One of the milkers had not showed up for work, apparently a common problem with him (his days were numbered) so we were short staffed to begin with. But between me and the head herdsman we worked our way steadily through all the cows and after a coffee break, we did those heifers that were at the main farm. I was easily finished by lunchtime for which I was grateful. It gave me a chance to recover from looking after my father the previous week, long days, and nights, his last at ever at home before he went into hospital.

I would appear early the next morning to do the youngstock which were in three separate places, two groups being needed to be brought in from grazing which I was told would take half an hour or so. Plus, we had to test the stock bulls. It went smoothly enough and again I had finished the test before lunch.

Reading would be on the Thursday and Friday mornings at a similar time. The milking herd went through easily, and the missing milker had turned up! So far, the test was clear, good news as the farm did have reactors in previous tests.

They thought there was no need to start so early on the Friday morning, we would soon get through the youngstock. I had arranged to meet up with one of my farmer friends for coffee at midday, I should be finished easily by then and after meeting up I could go into the office and submit the test online.

I arrived and we were ready to do a group of small calves not far away and while myself and a couple of the workers did these, the manager would get the bulls in. All good, we were soon done, and I texted by coffee appointment to say I had one hundred and ten heifers to do and would be finished, so should be on time to meet up. Nearly two hours later, two hours of total inactivity, I texted him again to say I still had one hundred and ten animals to do. My helpers had abandoned me to do something else. Was I frustrated, yes and quickly losing my patience. They did finally arrive where we were to test the last animals and it did not take long but I had been kept in limbo for far too long and wasn't happy.

But I had to bite my tongue and smile. A very frustrating last test to do and even when asked at a later date if I could help out again, the answer after this experience was a "No".

Taking an hour to test two animals, again frustrating and other people's patience may have gone, but I would also have to consider the funny side of it, watching or helping as the owners chased around the field trying to get their "herd" into a not very stable enclosure.

But through all those years testing, there were amusing times, frustrating times and as stated before, sad, and emotional times when you had to close down someone's farm because they had infected animals, ones that had failed their skin test.

At the end of the day, I could never lose my temper with the cattle, after all they would almost certainly rather have been somewhere else as well, and especially if on sixty day testing, the last thing they wanted was that strange man coming along and sticking two needles in their neck again.

A part of the job I will miss, certainly not. At times it has been amusing, tiring, hard work, frustrating. There are various other episodes of my testing described elsewhere. Some of the scares from it will remain with me forever.

Sadly, after all those years that I have been performing Tuberculin tests, are we any closer to eradicating this disease from the national herd. Sadly, the answer to that question is a firm no. It would be nice to think we develop a vaccine against Tuberculosis in cattle, in other infected species as well. It would be nice to have a better test for diagnosing it. At the end of the day, we work with what we have, far from ideal and we as cattle vets will soldier on in this eradication program.

But from now on, I will not be involved in that process although I do help a couple of farmers still with their tests, but from the other side of the fence, as the person getting the cattle in for the tester to test. From that, my joy of working with cattle can go on!

The emotions and stress the disease can cause in the farming community though is immense so perhaps now with that in mind, it is time to return to that topic of mental stress and wellbeing.

WELLBEING:

I HAVE ALREADY described scenarios where what has been going on at a farmer's workplace, on the farm, has impacted on him and his family. Certainly, David's herd going down with Tuberculosis just as he was about to sell the herd, and with the fact that he had made no winter provisions for the cattle, this would have impacted on his mental health, especially as he was such a good and conscientious stockman. Similarly with John and the loss of so many of his pedigree cattle through an inadvertent lead poisoning episode caused him and his family great mental strife. A life's work lost in such a short but devastating episode. The effects on the mental health of those concerned, in both cases was obvious to see in front of you.

To add to those cases there would be on many occasions when conducting TB tests on farms that you would have to tell the owners of cattle that the animal in front of you, when measuring the results of their skin tests, had failed, and would be classed as reactors. That meant they would have to be slaughtered and there would be a movement ban on cattle off the farm unless going to slaughter. Not only was there the mental impact of going down with the disease, but there was also the effect long term on management, having to keep calves which would normally be sold. Feed implications, cost implications and labour implications all adding to the mental distress of the farmer. Certainly, around where I worked, it got to the point of not if you got the disease on your premises, but when. The thought of the next routine test became more and more of a stress on all those involved. Sleepless nights and worry!

The stresses and strains of farming life were there for all to see. Those who may have read my previous books will know how much this subject of mental health means to me having suffered from it for so long myself, and I think having missed out on so much of the potential my life may have given to myself and to others while I suffered. I was lucky in that I found a cure for myself which gave me a new belief in myself that anything and everything is achievable if you are in the right mind to do so. So many wasted years before I found myself but in saying that I know how many other people suffer as well, some in isolation, others seeking help but still finding it hard to produce solutions. Sadly, there are still too many who cannot find an answer to their personal demons and sadly take the final solution.

Yes, a subject very much dear to my heart and which I have touched on in all my books, especially on my journey up Kilimanjaro where I did find my answers. In *"The Quiet Vet"* I have tried to describe some of the pressures that the modern vet, new graduates, young partners in veterinary firms, and farmers have to face, whether they be financial, work pressures or emotional. It seems to be the modern "disease" though putting that word in italics would be a misnomer, people suffering like I did myself those few years ago, shouldn't be classed as ill but deserve whatever help society can offer them so that they can fulfil their own potential, living in happiness and achieving all their goals.

Depression and mental illness can affect anybody, we are all candidates, so I wanted to explore where we are since I wrote last in *"The Quiet Vet"* on this topic in both the farming/rural community and my own chosen profession.

Jane and I were manning a stall at Minsterley Show in the summer of 2022, selling my book *"The Quiet Vet"* when we were approached a very well dressed lady who told us she was there to present an award to members of the rural community, and as it transpired one of the recipients was a farmer that I had close dealings with for many years in the Shrewsbury area. This was a Queen's Award for Voluntary Service, and it was going to be awarded to a group called Shropshire Rural Support.

What was their aim? It was in supporting rural people with confidential help reducing stress, risk of suicide and depression. I had been aware of support in the community from another farmer and had been to a couple of meetings which he had asked if I was interested in, but I thought this was more related to an organisation called *"Farm Community Network"*. I had attended a meeting where there were farmers, solicitors, land agents and other people involved in the farming community, and we were told about how to go about offering support to people we may be worried about in relation to their mental health and wellbeing. A talk was given by someone involved in the treatment of mental health but disappointingly to me I thought he concentrated on treatments (which we in attendance would not be able to give) rather than spotting the signs to look for in those that may be enduring a hard time, those people at risk.

I was interested to pursue what Shropshire Rural Support was about, especially as the start of it was initiated by someone I knew very well but I did not know his involvement in this. Clifford's interests were aroused some thirty years ago when he found out through the police that there had been twenty-seven suicides that year related to the farming community. This horrified him and he wanted to do something to try and reduce this number, offer some sort of network of support throughout the farming and rural community. Through his contacts in the NFU (National Farmers Union of which my father was heavily involved with many years ago) he found other likeminded people who wanted to help and support the community they worked in. Not many to begin with but they came from different parts of the community so that if they heard of a problem, it could be sent to the right person with the experience to deal with that particular problem.

I know from my own experience that if you are going through a bad time, and that may be financial, practical or emotional that you can isolate yourself away from your friends, the community that you live and work in. There had to be a way of reaching out to these people to offer appropriate help where necessary and support. It was important to spread the word that this support was available if only they could reach out and contact those people that were struggling with themselves and their lives. The group very much had the ethos that if you knew of someone who was struggling and potentially suicidal, then doing nothing was not an option and there had to be a mechanism that would allow for a member of the group to then approach this person to try and offer help and guidance. This can be a complicated process; I know when I suffered that I took myself away from other people and certainly did not want to talk about my problems with someone else.

But by offering this support whether by meeting and talking or just opening up pathways of communication the support group found that they were starting to help people and if there was an initial reluctance to accept this help, with the offer of regular communication then a lot of these barriers were broken down to the extent that help and advice was accepted and in a lot of cases lives were saved, depression and stress were reduced. There was a genuine appreciation that there were people out there who wanted to and were willing to help.

But what about them, the support group. They too were entering new waters and would come across situations that they had not met before, and may not have the experience to provide answers, solutions to the problems they were being faced with. Clifford became a great father figure for people to get advice from, but there was also a need to get some training from the people with real experience over many years in these situations, The Samaritans. They were extremely happy to offer help and advice, training as well to this band of rural supporters and some of them even joined them, staffing the phones for them at night to help people in other walks of life as well. They were gaining a lot of experience and were being able to use it in all communities.

But the important thing in all this was that in offering help that they also managed to keep their anonymity, there would be face to face contact plus their availability on the phone, but a first name was enough to give as a personal contact, and they would be careful not to divulge any other information about themselves or their family and background. They were offering support and did not want the "client" to become dependent on them despite that support they were giving.

What became important was to listen, and asking that question, "Are you fine" to which the usual reply would be "Yes".

But then the next question, "Are you really fine", and then being able to listen and notice any distress signs.

As the group grew in experience and became more well known, they needed a co-ordinator to organise the help where needed, to organise rotas for telephone duties so that there was always someone available at the end of a line through their confidential help line. But they also needed to raise funds to continue their work, to produce literature that they could hand out at local events, shows, the market, which people could take and if there was something that they related to, a problem, stress, depression then there was the link that they could follow up on, they had a contact.

So as a team they grew with a group of committed volunteers to deliver the service of rural support they wanted to give. They run as a charity but are always looking for volunteers to help in counselling, in fundraising, in marketing and PR, in events promotion, in finance and in IT. Why IT, because as we move into these days of smart phones and social media then as well as leaflets etc to spread the word of their existence and the help that they offer, more and more people, especially the younger generation look for the likes of QR codes that they can use on their phones.

Their role was providing a valuable service in our rural community in Shropshire and there were like minded groups being set up elsewhere in the country. There would be communication amongst these groups and that along with a national organisation that was set up, Farm Community Network (FCN). What these support groups could not offer was financial support, so often a cause of mental issues amongst the farming community where prices can fluctuate so much causing stress and what that can lead to. An example would be where you have stock to feed, but you are not getting an adequate return on your product, whether meat or milk (we have been through recent times where the pig industry has been a financial disaster), you have to feed your stock but may not have the capital to pay for that feed.

Another charitable organisation had been set up over 160 years ago, the Royal Agricultural Benevolent Institution which does offer further support along with practical and financial help and now aa 24/7 phone helpline. Members of these rural support volunteers could be members of both, even a Samaritan as well. The rural community is indebted to the time that these volunteers give up.

How do they spread the word that there are people out there to help and to listen. Leaflets, attendance at shows where they feel that they can't just put themselves out there as a stall saying if you need help come here, but have been innovative in their approach to attracting people, often isolated, by for example having a demonstration of old implements, tools that were once used on farms. People come to look, feel, and touch them, querying what they were and for what their purpose was. It gets them talking and through that a line of communication develops between them and someone who is willing to listen, and then willing to follow up that approach with further communication, the important thing being that if they say they are going to call or phone and at a certain time, they do so. The person with troubles must not feel that they have been let down, that their contact is there for them and will offer support if it is needed or they will find someone more suitably qualified who can offer more better advice for their needs.

Another important line had been through the Young Farmers Club organisations with volunteers often going to club meetings to talk about their role in the community. The high incidence of mental illness and suicide especially in young men is well publicized and here is a group, a generation in that risk category. In talking to an audience which they may reach out to young people with problems, and they may find suitable volunteers who can relate to this audience.

What is so important is that this rural support continues. The likes of Clifford have been acknowledged for their part in setting this up, but we all grow older and with that we have our own limitations. He has done his bit and deserves his rest from it now although he is still there to offer advice to other volunteers if needed, one cannot replace his experience and experiences. But it is just as important now that there is another generation coming in to continue this valuable work, not just in Shropshire but throughout the rural scene in the country.

An important question I had to ask was "Are things getting better?"

The number of calls to these help lines seems to be more complex .Is it a sign of the times, the number of calls seems to depend on time of year, the weather, lambing, calving, paperwork deadlines, family issues, Tb reading, succession planning, illness and isolation.

And the number of suicides? That is an interesting question that I cannot answer. But those support lines remain open and will continue to assist, give rural support to those that need assistance, to those finding life difficult, to those with emotional problems, to those who have lost someone dear to them and need help to get through tough times.

Through those early beginnings, the likes of Shropshire Rural Support have benefitted the local community and will continue to do so. They have received a prestigious award to honour what they have achieved. May they continue to do so while hopefully being successful in what they have made themselves available to do.

A very worthwhile group, giving their time freely to their local community.

I have found in my career as a vet that at times those wide-open spaces of the countryside, though beautiful, can be a lonely place. I could spend hours driving around between one call and the next alone with my thoughts or tuned into Heart FM. The isolation while waiting for the next call when we started working from home at the start of the Covid lockdown was daunting in that if work was quiet, you had no real contact with the outside world.

Farming, likewise, can be a lonely existence living in rural isolation. Living alone on your farm or with your partner and at times with no contact with the outside world. Hours working alone in the fields, on your tractor with nothing to think about other than the job at hand which you have done so often in the past that it is second nature, or stewing on problems in your life that are getting you down. An existence where you may live in a remote area or what contact you have with people is only that with your employees and increasingly these days, they are foreign and do not speak our language that well. A chance to talk or release your emotions becomes difficult.

But also, the very nature of the job is all consuming, occupying your mind and the majority of your time. You eat, you drink, you sleep (hopefully) and the rest of the time it is farming, farming, farming! Meeting some of these people at social events, at meetings then again if one engages in conversation with them, they talk about farming, what is going on back home. It is all consuming.

How many of these hard workers, when they come to retirement, find that they have no other interests other than what was their profession. Suddenly they have time to fill but no hobbies or pastimes to fill their time with. Some will continue to do "a bit" on the farm still if it is a family farm although their bodies are starting to be worn out, others just become lost with so much time to now kill. Mental strain!

But there are many farmers and their families who are again so occupied during their working lives that they do not have time or do not give themselves time to develop other interests. It is good that they can go to market once a week and meet other farmers and chat, at least it gives then at outlet for some form of communication but that is not the total answer for mental wellbeing.

I do feel that if they can develop other interests to take them away from their normal environment then that can only be of benefit to their long-term mental health. I have come across some in the community where I know they are struggling and have implored them to find other interests for their own good, something to give them a break from the lifestyle they live, farming is a commitment, a vocation. But there is only so much one can do other than make suggestions, it is then up to that individual to act upon the advice and pursue what may interest them.

In previous chapters I have mentioned that some people will be keen on sport, either playing it (especially rugby in these rural areas) giving them an outlet for a release of energy and a chance to meet other people, or becoming supporters, going to watch football or rugby. These sports have given me an opening to get to know some of the farmers better, to talk about something other than farming and have given the chance to release some of the tensions from the job that they do.

Others have found a release even on their own land, just by enjoying and appreciating what they have around them, nature. Walking, observing their hedgerows, the changing of the seasons and getting involved in conservation projects for the likes of protecting certain species (curlews would be an example of this in the area I have worked) or just trying to preserve meadowlands, a memory of the past that us older generation grew up in.

But what is important to me is that they for their own wellbeing, try to do something to give themselves an outside interest both to reduce their mental stress and to give them something to pursue when that day comes that they are no longer working, when they suddenly have so much time on their hands.

James, one of my farmers I had built up a working relationship with over the years would be a good example of this. He had moved down from Cheshire a few years ago and still had family roots up there. He had a successful three hundred cow dairy herd which was high yielding. I had collaborated closely with him trying to solve a lot of health issues on the farm and by enlarge, I think we had been successful. But two problem areas were arising. Firstly, as on a lot of farms, staffing was becoming a problem. He had a good herdsman but getting the continuity in support staff for him was getting more and more difficult. He and his wife were having to do more and more of the daily chores on top of what they had been doing in the past and this was impacting on their life. Secondly, the parlour was getting old and with that was creating problems in both the time it took to milk the herd, it was taking far too long, and with issues related to fluctuating vacuum pressures in the milking system, this was affecting the milking routine and udder health of the herd. We had talked through the issues and practical solutions, even getting milking machine experts in to try and come up with answers but it was looking to be costly and actually finding milking machine contractors to do what was necessary was proving impossible in the time frame needed.

Though he had a son and a daughter, neither of them was interested in carrying on the farm business though they did have jobs related top agriculture. After much heart searching, and with other health issues himself, James decided that this was the time to get out of the dairy industry. The decision was made to sell the herd and a date was set for a dispersal sale which soon approached very rapidly. A few cows were not suitable for the sale, and he would keep a while longer until he could sell them as barren. One or two who were too close to calving he kept and sold them as fresh calvers at the local market.

The herd was gone, and I rung him a few days later to see how he was. His daily routine had changed drastically from early morning starts and finishing whenever to a now more sedate life. But to begin with he was finding it hard to adapt away from a lifestyle he had become used to for years.

We had often talked after me doing my routine visits about one of our loves but with a bit of rivalry as he was a City fan, me United, football. He did when he could get upto the Etihad to support his team, something he enjoyed doing with his son. But it took the edge off it midweek getting home late at night after the game to have to rise early the next morning to do the milking. We also often talked about conservation, wildlife, the countryside in general.

It did not take him long to adjust to his new way of life with more of his time to do what he thought he enjoyed doing, he was now able to do it. As well as his main team he could go and watch the local team, Shrewsbury Town, and meet local people there. He now had time to walk around his farm watching the birds, the flowers, and the changing of the seasons. Had he packed up farming? No! He still had his land and was happy to sit on his tractor ploughing, rolling, fertilising, whatever job was necessary but the pressure on his time was gone. He was able to sit in the garden with his wife and listen to the birds sing. And, having been a livestock farmer all his life, after fattening and selling the beef animals he had retained after the milking herd had gone, he kept his hand in and his love of cattle by heifer rearing for a local farmer.

He had achieved a work/life balance that suited him now down to the ground. He had cattle on the farm, he could grow corn, continue farming his own land while now having the time to pursue his other interests.

Was I worried he would struggle to adjust, to have mental issues himself because I knew it was getting him down. Yes, I was, but we have kept in contact, and I am pleased to say that along with his other health issues now resolved, he is a happy and content man. He has been able to pursue other interests rather than stewing on the issues and worries of his farm. He has not needed outside support but has found his own solutions to a contented life and would now tell you that having enjoyed dairy farming for so long and having his own herd, yes it was what he had always wanted to do but now, selling the herd was the best thing he could have done at that time. A happy man.

Farming can be such a rewarding job but also can have its downsides both practically, financially, and emotionally. It is a job, it is a vocation, with many joys, comic moments, but also times that can be hard and moments that can be heart wrenching. At times it can be a much-maligned industry with urban communities thinking in a them and us mind, those that have and those that not. But farmers put a lot of time and effort into ensuring there is a food supply and into trying to maintain and develop the countryside in a positive way.

It is important that these rural support groups have developed and continue to support this vulnerable community. Everyone in the rural comm unity, in ant=y community for that matter, has a role to play in looking, listening for those that are struggling and then pointing them in the right direction, involving the support groups that are available so that they can provide the expert help that may be necessary.

Any potential suicide that can be prevented has to be a positive outcome. Hopefully through the work of these groups and us being the eyes of the comm unity, this positive outcome can be and will continue to be achieved. These people are out there for us, to listen and to help.

But what of my profession, so intricately linked to farming?

I have in *"The Quiet Vet"* described some of the pressures on the modern vet with the importance now of a work, life balance and the need for support for new graduates as they make their way into the world of being a qualified veterinary surgeon. I was interested recently to read an article that an ex-colleague had posted on Facebook worrying about the retention rate of veterinary graduates in the profession, saying a high proportion of these vets do not last beyond four years after qualifying.

Speaking from her heart she prefaced the article by saying "This is because our profession has to deal with so many crappy people that think they know better than vets, nurses and reception staff (they don't)." She adds "We have to put up with abuse, threatening behaviour and emotional blackmail every single day and there is jack all we can do about it, no wonder people are leaving the profession...and I'm so not scared to say it".

Words from a person who has worked in the profession for many years dealing with all aspects of modern practice. But does this underline some of the problems that we as vets have to deal with (other members of staff as well). A very honest statement from someone who cares about the line of work she has chosen to do and despite these feelings, has persisted with it.

She was commenting on a recent article she had read in "The Scottish Farmer" where on addressing an audience about the opening of another Vet School, university, in Scotland. A professor had quoted these figures of a high number of graduates only lasting in practice a brief time and saying these short retention rates needed to be addressed, stressing the invaluable role played by vets on the ground with farmers. Their role in sharing important disease updates and practical advice so critical to their farming profession. There was a thought that rather than producing more graduates, retention was more important as a sizeable proportion of them thought that their course did not contribute to the business skills needed. The preparation needed to work in a variety of high demand sectors including remote and rural practice was not happening. There was a need to attract students who already understood and appreciated the challenges and appeal of working in rural life (I guess I had that advantage in being a farmer's son and living away from my school life). These students would be better prepared to flourish in the environment they were about to encounter.

But this would have to go alongside better remuneration, and that subject I have mentioned many times, the work life balance. The modern graduate does not want to do the number of weekends and nights on call that I would have done throughout my career, the days of farm vetting being a vocation are disappearing. Or there must be better reward for working these antisocial hours, the changing expectations of the modern vet will need better recompense.

They are also having to deal with diverse ways of interaction and their respect coming from the emotional and challenging needs of their clients.

It is an evolving profession that needs to offer better support to graduates, and especially in rural practice may need to offer discipline specification to provide a mentally stimulating job and a focus to fully develop expertise.

So how is my profession coping with these changes in graduate demands, in working conditions, in mental wellbeing. I have already been through the mill, first suffering, then coping and finally overcoming depression. Part of this, but not all, was caused by the profession I worked in and some of its demands on me as a person. Because of my experiences, I have become acutely aware of the pressures on all that I have worked with and have tried my best to keep an eye out for others and offer assistance if I thought it necessary. I have become increasingly aware of the demands on us, and more importantly the signs of diminishing mental health in individuals in their day-to-day life.

Awareness is the key word here and is the direction I hope that as a profession we are now becoming more skilled in recognising key indicators of staff wellbeing and mental ill-health. I hope through my own personal experiences and further information that I have sort through courses and discussion, that along the way, then I may have been of help to some.

Through my travels after retirement, I met through a friend, a charming lady whose field of expertise was psychology, having worked in that field with both humans and animals. We chatted about my profession and the book I had just written, and she was especially interested in the chapter I wrote on mental health and wellbeing and was only too pleased to read it and give her comments.

She kindly did for me and read the chapter twice before making these comments.

"I am perplexed why (as you say) despite the often natural "calling" to be a vet, evolving from love of the countryside, working with animals, country folk and with the opportunity to mend and cure, your profession carries one of the highest suicide rates. Some of the difficulties that you mention a young vet can face seem identical to those men I worked with from other professions.

For example:

>*Long hours*
>
>*Disappointment*
>
>*Sacrificing family time for profession*
>
>*Financial worries*
>
>*Pressure/stress*
>
>*Business decisions, etc*

However, the difference, and I can completely relate to the personal responsibility and attachment to a living animal and empathising with the pure grief of its owner. I searched to see if any veterinary training was offered on how to deal with this personal aspect. There was a reason my profession expected us to study intense emotional empathetic feelings for 5 years! It seems you and your fellow students were given no emotional preparation and you were expected to work it out for yourself! I appreciated your account expressing the horrific supervising of the sheep and cattle and then having nowhere to share or debrief. I was sad to read Rod you had nowhere to work through these overwhelming dark feelings and instead had to sit through "jolly" dinner parties feeling completely alone and isolated. I am delighted to hear there are now developing rural support groups."

Perhaps this has just highlighted what I have said before, but interesting to hear it from someone outside my profession, someone who has had many dealings with mental health issues.

On of the things that came to the fore after my own problems was that I was not alone. With that, other people in the profession were starting to look at the problems amongst us and to try and find solutions, to provide help. In my last couple of years in practice, then there was a course of action to create more awareness of the issues in our own working environment, something that I was very keen to push. I went on some exceptionally good courses, others since have done likewise in courses organised by veterinary groups, but have they ticked the required boxes as necessary? From what I have been told, I have my doubts.

But during my last few months, we were distributed a card with a telephone helpline number on it. It was there if we needed it, if we felt we needed help. I think the trouble was that no-one really explained what it was or who they were, or what they did. Communication!

In looking to find where we are now, then I have taken a lot more interest in this helpline. So, it was of interest to me that soon after my struggles, there was a service set up to help us as vets deal with the pressures and stresses that we encounter in our day to day lives. Vetlife was set up in 2007 with the vision to support members of the UK veterinary community with high levels of physical and mental wellbeing. It set itself a mission to provide this support to the veterinary community and their families who have emotional, health or financial concerns whilst seeking to prevent such situations in the future. It strives to ensure that those engaged in the profession, the veterinary community, are aware of the sources of help and support should they, or a colleague, need assistance. Like the Rural Support Group, it points those individuals to additional sources of help as and when appropriate. That help may be short-term to help with an immediate crisis, or longer-term care for those affected by age, ill health, or disability, hoping to return those needing help to independence and self-sufficiency.

Like Rural Support, there is a helpline, contact by email and help will be provided by trained volunteers; vets, vet nurses and others with knowledge of the profession. An external supplier offers health support, and in some cases, financial support can too be offered.

It is a charity and so has high demands on financial resources with a fourfold increase in expenditure over the past fifteen years and is grateful for those who have undertaken significant fundraisers on their behalf.

An indication of what they now offer can be shown by their outcome and delivery reports for 2022, and even knowing the problems that my profession faces, I was staggered by the figures.

- Vetlife helped 3,503 contacts through its helpline, a 3% increase over 2021.

- Vetlife volunteers gave 18,750 hours of time to support the veterinary community.

- 216 contacts were referred on from Vetlife Health Support for psychiatric support, a 15% increase from the previous year.

- 44 applicants were helped through Vetlife Financial Support (236% increase on 2021).

Their work included expert led resources producing support in the veterinary community in "Loneliness" and "Suicide Postvention Guidance". Talks were provided to vet associations, vet employment groups and businesses to offer mental health support and to highlight the services they offer. Students in the nine vet schools were spoken to about wellbeing, plus the service visiting at key veterinary events.

The service is being widely used and is ensuring that there is an increased awareness in the profession at all levels, vets, vet nurses and support staff that there is help out there for anyone who needs it. Again, like Rural Support Groups, they are there to help, the message needing to be out there is that there is a service, Vetlife, that cares and is readily available to support the professions community if and when needed.

I am grateful to Vetlife for providing the information they have given me.

Another resource available to vets in this country, and they are now offering this resource internationally, is Mind Matters which is an initiative offered by the Royal College of Veterinary Surgeons. They aim to promote good mental health within the veterinary profession by offering a range of resources and training programs, including online courses, workshops and webinars. Started in 2014, their mental health awareness training has explored common signs and symptoms of mental ill-health, how to talk to someone who might be struggling, and how to effectively signpost. They have done this through promoting high-quality, evidence-based training and activities.

Despite its origins in 2015, I suppose, especially as one who has suffered from mental ill-health, that I would be disappointed that I knew little of this initiative until lockdown and Covid in 2020. At this time, then it did seem that Mind Matters did push themselves forward as a resource and have continued their education of veterinary staff and of students. But again, I would be disappointed that they state that only just over ten percent of those receiving training were rural vets.

It will be a resource that will continue to be developed, and I hope that the profession can engage with it. My worry is that it is a bit to theoretical, with the RCVS now offering grants for studies into mental ill-health, disabilities and chronic illness. They have introduced Mental health champions into practice from their training, but how many of those engaged in this are the senior management team. I for one, when suffering myself, would have chosen them as the last people to go to for help as some of the mounting pressures on me came from that very source.

It is a side that will continue to be developed, hopefully throughout all aspects of practice and training in this country. I hope that the new graduate coming into practice will in the future be far more aware of issues that they will face, and that there will be mechanisms in place to help them.

I was disappointed to hear from one former colleague now helping to manage a practice that when I asked her about how mental health was dealt with in her workplace, her reply was that no-one was bothered. This is an attitude that must change.

I hope in the development of a "more" team approach in my last workplace, that the barriers of them and us are broken down, that everyone working here becomes more aware of their fellow workers. Through this awareness, I hope that issues, warning signs of someone "in trouble" can be spotted early and they be signposted to someone who can help.

This will be an ongoing story in both the rural community and in my profession where it is a serious issue. It is obviously becoming more and more of an issue in all workplaces, but with our suicide rates in our profession, stepping in the right direction I hope points to a happier ending.

FIRST AID:

IT HAS NOT been uncommon in my past to have to explain what I actually did, what my job was. This was especially so to young children or when I have been abroad and there has been something of a language barrier. If I was struggling to explain, or not understood, then my fallback answer was always that I am "an animal doctor". That explanation was always clearly understood, though how often that was followed up by a question about what was wrong with the pet of the person you were talking to, whether it be horse, dog, cat, rabbit, or chicken. Nothing like a free consultation if you could get it. I did always have the get out clause that I was a farm vet, I did not treat small animals, though I would offer what advice I could.

Somewhere along the way, I was told that as a vet then we were allowed to treat humans, but the medical profession could not treat pets. I remember one incident, consultation, when I did do some small animal work that a medical doctor arrived in the consultation room with his young daughter and a cage. He explained to me that his daughter's hamster was in the cage, in its nest box and had not moved. They were worried and wanted to know what was wrong with it. I cautiously opened the cage and gently put my hand into the nest box to fetch the hamster out. Caution, yes because it would not be the first time that a dormant hamster would have bitten me. I retrieved this moribund pet, held gently in my hand ready for me to examine it. It was indeed very still, and although hamsters can go into hibernation, this hamster was obviously dead. I was going to have to break the sad news to this little girl, but was surprised that as a doctor, the father had not realised what the problem was, the lack of activity! He asked me if I was sure, and if there was a token gesture of placing a stethoscope on it, rigor mortis was the giveaway. I assured the medic that I was correct in my diagnosis. I wondered if he did know but wanted the vet to be the breaker of the sad news.

Certainly, in large animal practice, it would be common for a farmer to remark that they would be rather treated by a vet than a doctor. They would say that at least they would be seen the same day, like their animals were with any tests required being done straight away rather than having to be referred to a hospital. They would also often remark that our training as vets was longer but that is not true, as once qualified we are free to be let loose whereas a medic would do some sort of internship as a houseman to get more practical knowledge.

Farming and farm vetting can be a dangerous game, but in saying that one should not forget the small animal and horse vets confronted by snarling dogs, hissing cats and by nervous and unhand able horses, bites, scratches, kicks and many head traumas being a consequence of trying to examine these animals of a more than unfriendly disposition. I think in my few small animal days a dog may have bitten me once, kicked by an equine only once but it was a little Shetland pony so other than a bruise on the front of each thigh, nothing major. Cat bites, many times and you counted down the minutes before an abscess formed. Once when bitten through a fingernail I remember, and you could see the pus and gas building up under my nail. I had to drill a hole in the nail, painful but not as painful as the abscess would have been, to release these foreign fluids and gases from myself.

But as farm vets we deal with massive animals, bulls weighing well over a tonne in weight, over my career, cows have got bigger and bigger and still kick the same but with more force behind the blow. Sheep will generally run the other way, and it is only if you get caught below your centre of gravity as they run around that they may knock you over. Pigs, I would never trust them. Amongst them they are always inquisitive, sniffing, chewing about you as if you are some new toy to them. They are solid and strong, stubborn with a mind of their own. Their jaws are strong, their teeth powerful weapons. What was it I was often told, if you wanted to hide a body then feed it to pigs, they would soon destroy all evidence. On that happy note! But I would always be very conscious of their presence, on one of the welfare schemes we were supposed to inspect a proportion of the fattening pigs, go into their pens and walk around them looking for lameness, skin lesions, tail biting etc, signs of vice which could suggest their environment was not quite ideal. Some of these fattening pens although high enough to stand up in at the front, at the back of the sheds would be extremely low. One never felt happy stooping down so low while these inquisitive animals milled around you, nibbling your wellies, pushing and shoving their way around the pen. Somewhere along the line it was deemed a health and safety issue and we were allowed to observe from outside the pen.

But in my forty plus years in the profession I have seen and experienced myself enough injuries, but thankfully for me, no fatalities. They do happen on happen, and sadly to frequently. One hears of animals lashing out and breaking limbs, occasions where the handling facilities have been poor, a metal lever that operates the head lock on cattle crushes flying loose and hitting someone on the head, causing severe injury or death. There are many recorded incidences on farm of injury and death to the extent that in my final years, months as a vet, risk assessments had become an essential and necessary part of our job. If we were sent to do a Tuberculin test and we did not consider the handling facilities adequate, we were in our rights to walk away and say we would not do the test until facilities were improved. That never happened to me but certainly did to some of my colleagues. I hope that when issues arrived, we managed to reach some sort of compromise to ensure the safety of all those involved in doing the test. At the end of the day, it was our, as the vets there, responsibility to ensure the safety of everyone.

So did I escape Scot free, I wish, although thankfully I never received any major injury. Those days in Devon dealing with lame cows, a rope over the beam in the shippen, cow shed high above you then around the cow's leg, lifting the leg high so you could look at her foot. The leg and the head were the only parts of the cow secure, and the head not that well restrained so it was not uncommon for the cow to be hopping from side to side, leg held up by the rope, while you tried to support the leg you were examining on your knee, and she could lash out with it. The plus point was that if she did connect, you were so close to her that it would not hurt and, in those days, I wore waders which took away some of the impact of the blow. My early days in practice and perhaps things did not hurt as much as they did as I got older. Experience as time went by, I found ways of better immobilising the leg!

New, better crushes where automation took over from what we had before, and the introduction of specialist footcare technicians meant in my latter years, these blows did not happen. Seeing a lame cow, unless the technician could not fix her became very uncommon.

But have I escaped uninjured during all those years other than those kicks already mentioned. I wish! Even as long back as my days in Devon, when I was young and just starting out, I sustained my first injury. It was a kick but unlike most of them with a cow lashing out backwards, this was her kicking forwards between metal bars and catching me in the ribs with her toe. I think she knew what she was doing, her aim was perfect, in the process breaking one of my ribs. They are of course slow to heal and there is not a great deal you can do to aid the process, other than be careful. If I were to move a bit gingerly for a few days, it did eventually mend.

That was until a few weeks later in trying to catch a boisterous calf which leapt up as it went past me: snap, the rib had gone again and there would be another few weeks of grimacing in discomfort with any over physical exertion.

Surprisingly, I then went many years without any similar mishap. That is other than a serious car smash when someone went into the back of me, a whiplash injury which took months to get over and even now the effects on my neck have not gone away, and presumably never will. But that could have happened to anyone in a car, not just because I was a vet.

Tb testing, as I have said earlier, can be a hazardous task. I was up early one morning testing at Tim's dairy herd below The Lawley. We had finished the cows and would make a start on doing the calves at home before going onto his other premises where he reared the rest of his youngstock. There had always been a joke about one of his places where you could yoke the cattle's head with a lever either at the front or the back of the crush. I would be testing at the front end of the animal, Tim catching them from behind. If I did not watch out, as he pulled his lever down at the back, the one at the front also came down, sometimes hitting me on the head. In future tests he would put a tennis ball over the end of the front handle to reduce the blow to my head if it happened again, and it did.

But on this occasion as we started the calves, one trod on my foot, not the first time it had happened, and it certainly would not be the last. Why this time it hurt more than usual I do not know but it did! We finished the calves and retired to eat a nice, cooked breakfast before going on to finish the rest of the test. But over the course of the morning, I could not help thinking that my foot was getting increasingly painful.

At last, we had finished the test and it was time to wash down and take my boots off, but I could not. By now my foot was so swollen that the boot was going to stay where it was, on my foot. With a great deal of assistance, the boot was finally removed, and my foot was free but enlarged and bruised. Somehow, I managed to get a shoe on and return first back to the office, and then as I had started exceedingly early that morning, it was time to go home.

Shoe and sock off, I put my foot up to rest it. Lindsay, my girlfriend, came round later that evening. She was a technician in the ambulance service and on seeing my foot, decided I should go to A & E. For once it was incredibly quiet, we were the only ones there and as they knew Lindsay from her work, I was seen straight away and was soon having an Xray on my injured foot.

Nothing, no bones were broken we were at last told by the radiographer, but did I know about the three breaks I had had in my toes previously which were well healed. That was a surprise, some of those toes that had been trodden on in the past must have incurred more damage than this more painful incident.

But several of my veterinary colleagues, myself included as well, will have incurred injuries while Tb testing, especially to our hands while reaching through metal bars to either measure the cow's skin thickness or while injecting Tuberculin. Trapped fingers, very painful, especially as you continued testing with the injury, and once when my fingers were trapped between cow and metal, there was so much pressure on the end of one finger, it just burst, split open, and I could see all the blood collecting inside my rubber glove.

Another time, when testing again, a cow ran out of the yard and on seeing me tried to stop in her tracks. But there was dried cow muck on the yard, and it had just rained so it was very slippery. She could not stop, fell, and kept sliding straight towards me. I could not get out of the way and as she slid into me, I was knocked over backwards, falling, and catching my neck on a large concrete girder which was on the ground behind me. I felt stunned, and for a few seconds lost the sensation in my right arm before it returned with a strange tingling sensation throughout the limb.

Was the farmer concerned, not much, we still had over two hundred animals to do to complete the test. I continued, but again an injury which comes back to haunt me now and again.

Other than getting two back feet in my chest from a temperamental cow while trying to do a rectal examination on her, that was about it for me. Another broken rib, or more likely the same one broken again and experience by then should have told me that the cow could and should have been better restrained. We learn our lessons the hard way! But again, the farmer thought us hardy vets should just get up and get on with the job in hand. After all, he was paying for my time.

But we must not forget the farmers, they too get their fair

share of injuries, and often take the kicks that the cow had aimed at the vet, her intended target.

In all my years I have had three serious incidents where I did worry about the lives of the people I was working with, and it is not surprising that when talking about these, Tb testing is involved. Two of these incidents involve cattle panicking and running wild.

In the first, I was Tb testing with David, Paul, and their stockman down near the river in Shrewsbury. They had a group of cattle there for their summer grazing and they needed to be tested for Tuberculosis. A warm summers morning testing outside, getting groups of cattle into a coral, running them down a race into a cattle crush where I would test them and release them one at a time before moving onto the next one. We had one last group to get in, and this group was wild, nervous, and frightened. We managed to get most of the group into the yard and into the canal, and started testing this group, releasing those tested back into the field. We were nearing the end, left with just a few large beef animals and one of them was getting very worked up. She managed to escape and saw the exit route through the gate back into the field with her mates. She charged off towards them, but David was standing in the gateway. She was coming towards him. He was standing waving his arms and shouting hoping she would stop and return into the yard. She was having none of it and continued on her flight path which would take her right over David, she had no intention of changing course at all and ran straight over the top of him, knocking him off his feet and trampling over him.

This looked serious as he lay on the ground groaning. We reached him to find him starting to recover slightly and sitting himself up. A quick check over, he hurt but as far as we could tell nothing was broken, no limbs anyway. He was badly winded and much shaken, but otherwise said he was fine.

"WE must get her back in and finish the test," he said.

Bravado, yes, we did have to finish the test, but we would retire him to sit in a vehicle giving himself the chance to recover a little.

We did manage to get the animal back in and finish before

taking David back home. I rang later that day to see how he was, very sore and bruised. I had to read the test three days later and was not surprised to see David absent. It shook him and it was many days before he had recovered fully from the incident.

A similar incident occurred a few years later. A small suckler herd that I had attended for many years and knew from previous calvings and other visits that the cattle on this farm were wild. You did what you had to do and got out of the pen quick. The cattle were okay with John, the owner, but they did see him every day, they were used to him. Sadly, he was starting to show early signs of dementia but never seemed concerned about the presence of his cattle near him.

We were conducting his test because another neighbouring practice had said they would not because of the temperament of his cattle. I did the test helped by him, his wife and a couple of friends from a neighbouring farm I also went to.

It was going okay; we just had a group of large beef animals to do. We had to get them in a yard and then close a gate on them so that they could be filtered down into the cattle crush. But these cattle were big and strong and as we ushered them into the direction that we wanted them to go in, they turned and stampeded. Four of us in a line trying to stop them, but they charged forward towards the farmer's wife and ran over her. I rushed towards her hoping that I could save her, but realised if I did then it may turn even more of the cattle over her. They were gone and she was rolled in a ball on the concrete yard. Thankfully, because this could have been serious, again she was just badly bruised and shaken. Rolling in a ball and saved her from more severe injury as the cattle tried to step over her. Again, she was incredibly lucky in what could have been a fatal incident.

The cattle were too wild, too uncontrollable and as John's dementia deteriorated, we managed to persuade him that these cattle needed to go before there was a significant injury. It was his life, his cattle, but here it was getting too dangerous.

Health and Safety was becoming increasingly essential in

these environments, the risk assessments necessary, and with the increasing reports of farm injuries and fatalities nationally, it was decided that we as vets should start undertaking some sort of First Aid training. We started as a practice running courses where we would attend along with any farmers who wanted to subscribe as well. A trained paramedic would come and run the course, going through the most likely injuries to occur in our workplace, how to recognise symptoms of stroke, heart attack etc, going through CPR and then wound and limb a management in the case of injury.

I do not know why but I always seemed to end up with Jill as my practice partner for Heinrich's manoeuvre, bandaging up and CPR with our plastic dummy, Annie. We are good friends!

In time all vets and support staff were trained First Aiders, along with many of the farms who would send a member of staff along to the courses. The first was very good, the second as we renewed our training every three years, I don't know, was our trainer having an off day, it was not a good course, and everyone got a refund from it.

My final course was during Covid, I was supposed to go with two of the other vets to a training centre in Stoke (we would all go in turn) but lockdown came along and it never happened. In the end we did it online, in small groups in Zoom meetings. The instructor was excellent, enthusiastic and the more questions you asked him, the more he warmed to his task. The difference with this course was that we would have a practical as well when lockdown allowed and would have to pass a test to have our First Aider status acknowledged. We did this in pairs, observing social distancing, bandaging various plastic limbs, working defibrillators, and again having to demonstrate a competence with CPR.

I guess the only time the courses came in use for me practically was not on farm but when I was out walking one night when home from work and a motorcyclist was hit by a car behind me. Someone had to take control of the situation until an ambulance arrived with the biker knocked off his bike and sprawled out on the road. My practical training came in useful in this situation, though when

I said to the surrounding audience that I was a First Aider and a vet, I do not know how they saw that, this was not an animal we were treating. The ambulance came, police took statements, and I finished my walk.

But the time I really needed this training was an incident that occurred on farm before these courses were instigated.

A sunny summer's afternoon would take me to Bill's to look at a lame cow and to pregnancy diagnose some heifers that had got in with the bull but should not be in calf.

The lame cow came first, a front foot to look at, never the easiest if it was not a good cattle crush. She was not happy we wanted to look at her foot, restrained in the crush with a head lock and a metal bar behind her so she could not move around too much. I lifted her foot and secured it to a block of wood intended for such use and started pairing her foot to find the cause of her discomfort. I had nearly finished, but s one gets closer to the sore point it obviously becomes more painful. She struggled and somehow managed to knock the metal bar forward with some force. It hit me on the head, and I would have to say that I did not feel too good but completed the task in hand before releasing the cow and taking a minute or two to regain my composure.

I think I was slightly concussed. Bill of course was keen to continue, us vets are hardy chaps and a knock to the head was nothing!

The next task was to pregnancy diagnose the group of heifers and to inject any that were in so they would abort the foetus, they were too young to be carrying a calf. We had to get the group in from another yard and into a pen behind the crush where we had been examining the lame cow. The lad who was helping us drove them through the yard and towards the pen they had to go in, Bill and I waited behind a solid gate which we would close behind them when they had passed us. They went into the pen then panicked and started to rush towards the yard they had just come from. Bill and I had started to close the gate behind them. But as they turned and rushed back out again, the gate was forced back, with Bill and I trapped between this and the wall behind us, being pressed against the wall with some force as a few tonnes of prime beef ran past. It did hurt, but as Bill let out a groan, I thought nothing more of it other than him being winded by the force of the gate, he had slightly less room than I did, and I felt a bit battered.

We were going to have a rethink on how we were going to get the cattle back again when looking down a noticed a patch of blood appearing on one of Bill's trouser legs.

What had happened?

The metal gate was hinged to its post by a large bolt which had a long free end the other side from the hinge, and with a wide thread so a nut could secure the hinge tightly onto the gate. At some stage this had become bent, so sticking outwards and with the force of the cattle running past this bolt had penetrated Bill's leg into his thigh.

We needed to examine this further and by now he was feeling a little faint and was looking very pale. Taking an arm each over our shoulders, our helper and I managed to get him outside into the sunlight where he could rest against a wall. The bleeding was getting more profuse, we needed to get a proper look at this wound.

I had to remove his trousers down to his underpants. I did not think this was in my job description, but....it had to be done.

There was a sizable puncture wound in the leg, which was bleeding, but the blood flow did seem to be slowing down. I told the helper to look after Bill while I went back to the car to get some bandages and a tourniquet, we had to stop the bleeding. It did look as if this would need more than just our medical attention so when I got back to the patient, I got the helper to go and call an ambulance, either from his mobile if he had any reception or ring from the house.

I applied a tourniquet to stem the flow of blood and then applied a pressure bandage over the wound and around Bill's leg with the equipment I had got from the car. He did look slightly perkier now, but he was in some discomfort.

There seemed to be no sign of blood now coming through my

bandage, so I was able to start releasing the torniquet gently. His trousers were down around his ankles, we would have to complete the job and remove them totally, leaving him bare footed with a nice white bandage on one thigh, otherwise just standing there in his white pants. Not the prettiest sight I have ever seen.

But as he started to feel more comfortable, we managed to manoeuvre him around to the other side of the buildings where we could sit him down while we waited for an ambulance to arrive. We were in the middle of nowhere so were not expecting a rapid response. His wife did come back from town, and we were able to give him a warm drink tea with plenty of sugar to help him. Otherwise, it was just a wait, keeping an eye on his colour and his general demeanour.

Eventually, and they were as quick as they could be, an ambulance arrived and we were able to tell the paramedic what had happened, when and what we had done.

My bandaging of less than an hour ago was cut loose and the wound examined. It had stopped bleeding, but one could see a gaping flesh wound, now bruising quickly. The edges of the wound were quite rough.

Having done their assessment of Bill, the ambulance crew redressed the wound and loaded him into the ambulance to take him into A & E. We were left to tidy up our discarded bandages etc. His wife asked if we were going to carry on and finish what I had come to do.

We suggested that with Bill's leg and my head that enough was enough for the day. She reluctantly agreed.

I obviously wanted to be kept informed of his condition. He was admitted and the true extent of the wound was discovered. It transpired that it had been lucky that the penetration had been a traumatic entry by a jagged instrument, the hinge. It had penetrated deep into the thigh, through the muscle mass and coming very close to the Saphenous artery. There was a lot of damage, and it was touch and go for a few days as to whether the blood supply to the lower limb had been permanently impaired.

Could he lose the leg?

It was a worrying few days before at last good news, as the healing process got under way there appeared to be some revascularisation of the leg, the Saphenous artery seemed to be functioning again, and after a suitable time of recuperation, Bill could return to a normal life. It did take a long time but thankfully when I see him these days one would not know that there had been this risk, of losing a leg, he seems perfectly normal.

A freak injury which could have serious long-term consequences for Bill, but it just underlines what dangers can be around the corner on farms, and what some basic knowledge in first aid can do to help in these situations.

These accidents are infrequent, but they do happen. Okay, kicks and knocks usually cause some bruising but that soon wears off. How many times has my head come in contact with a cow's heavy head as she swings it about while being restrained. Cattle get bigger and stronger, with that our workplace must become a safer place. We have to be more aware of possible dangers.

Should I have driven back to the office from Bill's when I almost certainly had a mild concussion. The safe answer, NO.

I am out of the battlefield now, but one hopes in the future that the number of these incidents lessens, and the farmyard becomes a safer place.

Now, even in retirement, I shall try and keep up to date with my first aid, you just never know when that knowledge may be needed, and it may help a life be saved.

AFRICA, SAMOSAS, and a LIFETIME'S DREAM:

ANYONE WHO KNOWS me will know of my love for this continent and East Africa, with its mountains and game reserves especially. Ever since childhood the continent has held a fascination for me, with a powerful desire to visit which has persisted through my life. There was an ambition to climb Kilimanjaro, the highest mountain on the continent, the "roof of Africa" by the time I reached my fiftieth year, but somewhere my life got side tracked through bringing up a family and then with the effects of depression. I passed fifty and the best I had managed was to view the distant shores of North Africa from Gibraltar. I had failed in my ambition and had resigned myself to the fact that what had fascinated me for so long on the grasslands of the Great Rift Valley, I would never get to see what I had so much hoped for.

In 2011 I did manage with Jane to get to Egypt with a trip, a cruise down the Nile. If not the East Africa I had so longed to see, at least I had now stepped foot on this great continent. And with that I suddenly found an interest in the history and culture of this once great civilisation who traded deep into the heart of Africa on this long river. Egypt was fascinating, a new experience for me but had not satisfied that lust to go on safari or to stand at the top of the continent. With that, depression which had been creeping up on me for a number of years now overtook me as I plunged into dark places. But it was on this cruise that I found a little poem, just a few lines of prose which gave me the inspiration to realise that it would be me and me alone who would overcome this mental illness. I slowly started taking steps towards a better and more enlightening future, I was about to be reborn with a purpose in life and goals that I had never had before.

If that little poem gave me a direction, then the thing that really changed my life was at last, even at the age of fifty-eight, a chance to climb that mountain. A plan but then still lacking confidence in myself, I found many reasons why I should not do it, this trip which was now arranged. For every reason I came up for backing out, two friends especially produced counter arguments of why I should do it. On July 5th, 2012, I stood on the roof of Africa, I had succeeded in that lifelong ambition and have never looked back since. How climbing one mountain, Kilimanjaro, could have such an effect on one's life I do not know. But it did and gave me a new perspective in life, a confidence I had never had in myself before and a will to succeed and fulfil more ambitions.

I had promised when looking up at the peak from below when back at our hotel the following day that I would return. I had climbed the mountain but what about all that wildlife, other than a few monkeys on our way up, I had seen nothing. I promised myself that in five years' time I would be back and would safari. I would at last see the Serengeti, Ngorongoro and the great plains that were the habitat of all those species of wildlife I had for so long wanted to see. David Attenborough films are great, but they are different from seeing these wonderful beasts in the flesh.

Those five years passed, and an ever more confident Rod fulfilled his promise to himself but this time visiting Kenya, firstly to climb Mount Kenya, the second highest mountain in Africa and then to visit the Masai Mara, Nakuru and then Amboseli and at last see an elephant, many elephants, in the flesh.

My stories of those trips are recounted in *"Kilimanjaro. My Story"* and *"Kenya. A Mountain to Climb"*, books which I thoroughly enjoyed writing on topics dear to my heart.

But another purpose of the Kenya trip was to raise money for the charity *"Send a Cow"*, I had been lucky enough to be selected to go out the following year to Kenya to help in a project the charity was running where vets would go in pairs for a fortnight and teach charity representatives on the ground from there, Rwanda, Burundi, Ethiopia, Uganda and Zambia better livestock management and productivity so they could then go and spread the word to local small holders. We hoped to try and reduce poverty, improve nutrition, and give more hope to the future as well as encouraging female empowerment.

And so, it was after an enjoyable trip in 2017 to Kenya, I would return the following year in May 2018, but now with a purpose to impart my knowledge to this willing audience. Before Kilimanjaro and the old Rod, there is no way I would have had the confidence in myself to do this but now, along with my colleague, Anna Patch, I would do something that in the past I thought myself incapable of, teach an unknown audience.

I left England on a bright, sunny day, it would transpire that we would not see any rain for weeks. Catching an early train out of Telford, I caught a train to London then Heathrow where I would meet up with Anna. She was travelling up from her home in the West Country. We had met once before but only very briefly so we had a couple of hours to kill at the airport getting to know each other before boarding a flight to Nairobi in Kenya, and then a short internal flight to Kisumu having met up with our co-ordinator from *Send a Cow*, Sheila Halden. Then it was a couple of hours by car, stopping for breakfast on the way before arriving at our destination near Busia close to the Ugandan border. I had been travelling for over twenty-four hours by the time we arrived at the convent which was the site for our course over the next few days. Anna and I had briefly discussed our agenda for the next few days while on the plane but did not get very far as we thought it best to meet up with Sheila for her to explain exactly what she wanted from us.

Having settled into our rooms, we met up with other members of *Send a Cow* Kenya to discuss our timetable, visits arranged to local farms where we could put our teaching into practice before visiting the attached farm to see what practical aids we could use from there. Sadly, we witnessed a very distressed cow who had prolapsed her uterus earlier in the day and was in a bad way. If in England, I would have put her out of her suffering, but here all we could do was make her more comfortable and hope nature would work a miracle. Unfortunately, she died over night.

The clouds were gathering by late afternoon, and we would soon be experiencing what it is like when it does rain in the main Kenyan rainy season, it chucked it down but luckily, we had just got back to our accommodation before the rain got serious.

Over the course of the evening, having experienced the very temperamental plumbing system, you may get a hot shower, a cold shower or just a few drips depending how it felt, we joined up with the group of people we would be working with. The nine or ten we were informed we would be lecturing turned out to be sixteen. Did I find that a bit more daunting? I suppose yes but we would get on with it and give it our best go!

The following morning after breakfast we met up with them all in the classroom, introducing ourselves properly and telling them more about our background and our previous visits to Africa. Then it was time to get into our program under way with a rather reluctant audience to begin with, trying to get them all to participate in our early teachings. Luckily, there were two or three who had been on previous courses who were extremely willing to help us get things moving. A trip to the farm that afternoon broke down more barriers as we were able to talk to everyone on a one-to-one basis, and that started our daily routine of a morning in the classroom and an afternoon on a farm, a different one every day.

Day two took us to a farm near Lake Victoria where we would deal with our chosen subjects, donkeys, and goats. We managed to combine our knowledge along with two of our students who collaborated closely with a donkey charity to teach enough about donkey husbandry and welfare but were still struggling to get much audience participation.

I was rather horrified to be given for my lunch what looked to me like deadly nightshade, and that is what it was but on pointing out it was poisonous, I was assured that when boiled twice it was quite safe. I am still around to tell the tale! But I suppose that is how any resource can be used even if to me it was tasteless. We had a long drive back to the convent, experiencing yet another downpour which had closed the road in places but did not affect our route back. We would pass near the village where Barrack Obama's grandmother lived, a local legend. We would hear his name later our trip!

Anna and I thought we were making progress with our agenda and slowly but surely were getting our students to think the way we wanted them to about husbandry and especially about communication, so that they could then go out and spread the knowledge we had given to them. But what we both wanted was to break down the nationality barrier, to be able once we had come out of the classroom to meet them on equal terms, not as teacher and student but just as adults meeting up for a chat in the evening. One or two of them, especially Fanuel who referred to himself as a "real man" were great, but they usually disappeared into town in the evening for a drink, the others departed straight after our evening meals to their rooms leaving Anna, Sheila and I to sort the next day's program out. We would have loved to have joined them in town.

Our fourth day, we reversed the routine doing the farm visit first before coming back to reflect on what we had learnt that day. That would mean taking a packed lunch with us on the coach which the kitchen had prepared for us. I was surprised up to then at the appetite of everyone on the course though I was struggling with what was served up every day. I love eating fish but only have to find one bone for it to put me off the rest of the dish. The fish from Lake Victoria had plenty of bones so were a non-starter for me. The lovely ladies in the kitchen noticed my appetite and did start cooking little things just for me, bless them.

After our farm visit that day, concentrating on poultry which luckily Anna knew far more than I did, we went back onto the coach to have lunch then drive back.

The kitchen ladies had done us proud, fruit, drinks and two boxes of samosas to eat between us, and they were delicious and everyone when back on the bus had their fill. We were ready to depart back to the convent, well fed and happy. Anna and I sat near the front of the bus, Fanuel just opposite us and most of the ladies on the course just in front of us. The men, as they do, occupied the back few seats and everyone was thinking of getting a bit of shut eye while on the way home.

It seemed a shame for all those remaining samosas to be going to waste. Anna came up with the bright idea of betting Fanuel that he could not eat them all before we got back to the lecture theatre. Twenty-five dollars was on offer if he could succeed and he was extremely happy to accept the challenge, it would be nothing to a real man! We counted the samosas, thirty-eight in total remained in the box so Fanuel had about a hundred minutes to eat them before we got back.

Word spread through the bus, and if nothing else we had broken the ice and had everyone, especially the men in good voice and chatting continuously to us. He had soon acquired a manager, an agent, and a coach as he started on what he thought would be a simple task. He would eat them all and then have a quick sleep before we got back.

Many conversations began on the topic of whether he would succeed, the men a definite yes, the women erring on the side of caution, Anna confident she would come out on top and myself more than a little unsure which way our wager would go.

The box of samosas was placed on Fanuel's lap, and he began his task, the first one picked up then one bite, and then a second and it was gone, a minute no more and any sign of it had disappeared. Perhaps it was an easy task, now only thirty-seven left to go. Over the next quarter of an hour, with plenty of encouragement coming from the back of the bus, manager, coach, and agent all offering much vocal support, one by one the samosas were starting to disappear. Fanuel was enjoying his food and enjoying the thought he was going to make an easy twenty-five dollars.

Anna was still confident; I was now erring on the side of Fanuel succeeding. The samosas were disappearing nearly as quickly as the miles!

Fifteen were gone, the guys in the back counted them often enough to be able to give a running score, but now were there signs of a little slowing in the rate of consumption? They were still being eaten but certainly not at the rate of earlier in the journey. Now we were at twenty, and there were signs of just a little bit of confidence draining away from our real man. Each samosa's journey to Fanuel's lips seemed to be taking longer, each bite slower. Our man was starting to struggle and was now starting to sweat profusely. But we ensured he also had a bottle of water in his hand so that he drank plenty as well.

Twenty-one, twenty-two, twenty-three. They were slowly going one by one, and if there was still a strong look of determination on his face, Fanuel now looked like he was struggling a little. But he had a bet to win and with his supporters in full voice egging him on, he was not going to give up.

Slowly but surely, they were eaten, and he was not going to stop despite the ladies in the front saying it would not do him a lot of good and that he should stop.

We were down to ten and now less than half an hour from base. It was obvious our driver was following events in his rear mirror, and probably not in the rules, he stopped by a river to let everyone out to stretch their legs, all except Fanuel, Anna and I. Was this a ploy to give him more time so that the local hero could win the bet against us "foreigners"?

We were all back on the bus again, the last leg of the journey and the end of the box of samosas in sight. Slowly, and it was slowly now that each samosa disappeared down Fanuel's throat, smaller bites, more chewing, and more sips of water. I guess at this stage I really wanted him to stop because as time wore on, he looked increasingly uncomfortable.

Fifteen minutes left and down to five and the rate he was

eating them, Anna knew she was now on to a winner. But was the driver now going slower and slower, yes, he was. We knew whose side he was on!

Four left, another big drink of water and Fanuel was now sweating a great deal.

"Stop now before you are ill," the ladies implored.

But with grim determination he soldiered on, three left then two. But time was now running out. It took him so long to eat each one that he could not possibly succeed in his task. One more down and one to go as we entered the driveway of the convent. He would have to have eaten it by the time we went through the gates. The crowd was going wild, willing him on to succeed and with that he started on the last one, eating as fast as he could but by now it was painful to watch him eat so slowly.

The gates approached; the samosa was gone. Fanuel had succeeded, had won the bet, and Anna handed over his reward, well deserved.

But as we pulled up outside the convent it had reached the time something had to give. Fanuel stood up, lunged to open his window, and sticking his head out before the bus came to a halt, he was violently sick, all down the side of the bus. That will teach the driver to have slowed down!

We adjourned to the dining room for a quick coffee before we would start on the days lectures, reflecting on what we had seen at today's farm and now with a more than willing audience participation, especially from our Rwandan representatives who were more versed to working and advising on poultry, a couple of them had their own small flocks. There was one noticeable absentee, Fanuel was nowhere to be seen, having retired to his room. He did have the room next door to me.

During the course of our class discussions, I did wander to the back of the classroom and looked out of the window down onto where the bus had been parked. The driver was now frantically brushing the side of the bus Fanuel had been sick down, and if the gods were on his side, it was time for our daily downpour, far more powerful than the driver's hose to aid him with his cleaning job.

Fair play to Fanuel, he did return for the second part of lectures, though looking far from one hundred percent, and did appear for supper. His appetite had returned. A "real man"!

Anna and I had at least broken the ice with our pupils now and we chatted freely about anything and everything whenever we could. But we still wanted to break that barrier that we may get invited into town, into Busia, with some of them to share downtime with them in their own environment. The weekend was approaching and we still had a lot of work to cover so to allow as many as possible to go on an excursion on the Sunday, we decided we would have to continue our teaching on the Saturday morning starting early so that if we reached where we wanted to be, everyone could go off in the afternoon and then have a complete break on the Sunday. We had reached the stage where we wanted to put everyone in the position that we were in, they were now the teachers as they would be when they would go out to smallholders, those who wanted to participate in the *Send a Cow* project. We started with the experienced members giving them a topic we had covered, and the rest of the class would be their audience. They had to be able to communicate the messages we had given to this demanding audience. We sat at the back of the class and at the end offered criticism or praise as to how each Pir had done in their presentations. One or two of the class made excellent awkward farmers.

We were done well before lunch, class dismissed until Monday morning. What was everyone going to do now, they were heading off in groups into town, into Busia. Anna and I asked a couple of them what they were going to do, hoping we may get an invite to join them, but none were forthcoming. We resigned ourselves to enjoying the sunshine (until our daily storm arrived) reading in the grounds of the convent. There we sat as everyone disappeared off down the drive leaving us by ourselves. But two of them stopped, came back, and asked us if we would like to join them.

We of course jumped at the opportunity, "We would be ready

in five minutes."

Harisa and Emelda waited for us, he Kenyan and she the Zambian amongst the group, and then we set off towards the main road. We found the rest of the gang also waiting there trying to get a lift on these wonderful minibus forms of transport they have in Africa, where if there is a space, even outside the vehicle, someone will be hanging on to it. We did not seem hopeful of getting a lift so walked down the road to the bus stop before. A small queue but it was not long before we were on board a bus and travelling towards Busia, passing the rest of the gang still waiting.

What we did find was that our US dollars which we were told to bring with us from home, they were used everywhere, would not buy us a bus fare. Harisa paid for us, we would have to find a money exchange in Busia so we could pay him back and offer some hospitality to our hosts when surely eventually we would find ourselves in a bar.

The bus was nearly empty, us four near the back and probably half a dozen Kenyan men near the front. They kept on turning and looking at us and then going into deep conversation with each other. It was very disconcerting, was it because of our colour and a resentment from former times of British colonial rule? We did not know but felt uncomfortable as this continued as we ate up the few miles between the stop and our end of journey in Busia. Eventually we asked Harisa to ask them what was going on. He went to the front of the bus and started a conversation with them often turning and pointing at me.

He came back up the bus to us with a smile on his face. If I had mentioned earlier that Barack Obama had family connections, some of his Kenyan roots in this south-west corner of the country, then for some reason these gentlemen on the bus thought that I was his brother.

Surely not, I do not look like him and I am not even the same colour but that is what they thought, and they were not changing their opinion. Their looks, glances back, continued until it was time to get off the bus and find a money exchange.

Somehow across the square, the rest of the gang had arrived at the same time.

An interesting journey and how I played on my now notoriety, the brother of the former head of the free world, and now here in Busia!

Busia is a town bordering both Kenya and Uganda, a busy throughfare having parts in both countries with a main route through to Nairobi from Kampala, linking the two capitals. We needed to change some of our dollars into Kenyan currency so asked Harisa where we could do so on a Saturday afternoon. He was local and knew just the place to go, which just happened to be near the border point. Anna went first, exchanging a hundred dollars, then me doing likewise but I am sure her good looks got a far better exchange rate than myself, even if I was Obama's brother.

What to do now. Emelda wanted to buy a dress, not quite what I had envisaged doing on a weekend in Kenya, but I would go with the flow. Harisa said follow him, he knew just where to go and promptly led us straight across the border into Uganda.

Anna and I were a little apprehensive, asking "What about passports, visas etc?" Which we did not have with us anyway.

"No. Don't worry," said Harisa, "It is nothing to worry about."

We strode on into Uganda. By my count, three of us were aliens and had just walked across an international border unchecked. Yes, we were a little worried. We continued down the main street looking for the dress shop Harisa knew of. Goats with bloated stomachs grazed the roadside eating anything and everything they could find. We at last found the shop but there was nothing suitable here, but the owner had another shop just up the street, and here Emelda, with Anna's approval, found the dress she was looking for. She tried it on gaining all our approval, and then with a little bartering it was hers. We continued on our way, Anna, and I still more than a little concerned about our presence in this country.

Harisa pointed out the rest of the gang walking the other side of the street.

He said, "They stand out far more than us."

How could that be? There may have been a few of them, but in our small group of four were the only two whites to be seen anywhere! We felt conspicuous, very!

We decided it was time for a beer and so left the main street, disappearing down a street to our right lined with bars and many streetside barbeques where chickens were being roasted on spits, ready for any passers-by like us to feast upon them. But we wanted a beer, not a chicken.

We found a bar and some empty seats where the four of us sat and waited for a waitress to appear. This is where we found out what a friendly nation we were in, even if everyone who were only too keen to speak to us, though in Uganda, were in fact Kenyan. A massive bloke opposite started to talk to me, and we were soon on that universal language, football. It seemed everyone here was either an Arsenal fan or a Man Utd fan. My new friend, like me supported Utd. Not the most exciting conversation for Anna to enjoy but it was nice to talk to a local and his family, he had his kids with him as well.

It was getting to that time of day again, and as I looked out of the bar window the skies were getting blacker and blacker. Oh, the joys of the rainy season, but at least we were inside, and looked like being so for a little while. Lightening lit up the skies, sheets of it, and with that we lost all power. We sat there patiently in the dark waiting for power to be restored. Luckily, the bar had its own generator, but then the heavens opened. Chickens disappeared off the street at whatever stage of cooking they were at, and we watched the rain cascading down outside in the gloom of early evening in the rainy season. I guess it was time for another beer and more talk of football until the rains abated. Anna was content, she was now on G and Ts.

At some point I needed the loo and made my way in that direction, passing the main bar on the way. There sat an attractive and buxom lady, who as I passed reached out and gave my backside a large squeeze. A smiled and walked on, taking this as some sort of Ugandan handshake! The loo, no lights, and no lock so it was a matter of pointing in what one hoped was the right direction while trying to keep one foot firmly against the door.

At last, the rains abated and having supped up we decided it was time to go, time to find something to eat though it would be a chicken. What was a dry street when we entered the bar was now a muddy passage interspersed with deep puddles. No streetlights yet, so we tiptoed through, around the puddles using the torch on a mobile phone to find our way. And somewhere on that muddy path we crossed back into Kenya, I am not sure where. We felt relieved but could tick off another country visited.

The four of us found a nice club to have a meal before getting a taxi back to the convent. But we were late, and if Anna and I thought there may be overtures of romance between Harisa and Emelda, it was soon cut short when Harisa found he was locked out of his room and would spend the night sleeping in the storeroom, an open door he could find. It had been an enjoyable, an interesting day and we had thoroughly enjoyed their company. It turned out the rest of the gang ended up in the same bar, owned by the brother of one of them.

Our exploits of the day, the evening soon spread amongst the rest of them, and for *Send a Cow's sake*, we hoped there would be no repercussions from our illegal entry into another country. Thankfully, all was laughed off and we had broken down all those barriers.

It had in the end been a fun day, at last getting out with some of our new African friends to enjoy some of the local life. An interesting experience, firstly on the bus, crossing the border and enjoying a very pleasant time in the bar with Kenyans, and finally a nice meal on the edge of town, but firmly in Kenya.

The next day was going to be our excursion out. Initially, Sheila had asked Anna and I if we fancied going to the Kakamega forest, she was a very keen bird watcher, and the forest offered the chance to see many species (367 if you were that lucky). We could get a hotel on the Saturday night so we could have a full day in the forest. We were keen but also wanted the chance to go out with the others on the Saturday which we eventually did. So, we opened the trip up to everyone on the course and surprisingly they all wanted to go, so we arranged to go by bus straight after an early breakfast. This was our rest day, but we hoped that there would be something to gain by observing nature at work, how different ecosystems managed to work side by side offering diversity and survival.

The Kakamega forest is a tropical rain forest, the last of which to survive in Kenya, and is Kenya's last remnant of the massive ancient Guineo-Congolian forest that spanned much of the continent. It is elevated between 1500-1700metres above sea level but has several water courses that feed eventually into Africa's largest lake, Victoria.

We were greeted there by a couple of Park Rangers who would guide us, split into two groups through the forest explaining some of its ecology but also pointing out its fauna and flora. A forest with an abundance of bird species. Trees, some of which only exist in this forest, plants, insects, animals which would mainly be monkeys, but hopefully we would not come across the various species of poisonous snakes that frequented the lower canopies of the forest.

The forest has an exceedingly high rainfall but as we set off on our walk it was sunny and dry. It was a fascinating walk as our guide led us through well-trodden paths pointing out this plant and that. But what was fascinating was the vast amounts of information about some of the medicinal properties that these plants had, widely used by the local "witch doctors". One would be fascinated to know what success they had as our guide even suggested that locally some of these plants had been used as treatments against certain types of cancer.

It certainly made you think that there should be openings for research into these local medicines and their benefits. Enlightening, most definitely it was.

Our walk took us up a hill where the forest opened out into grassland, and on reaching its peak we were rewarded with the most fantastic views over the forest, its water courses and far beyond. What a pleasure it was to stand and view over this vast expanse of rain forest and to the parts of Kenya which were beyond.

It was time to descend back into the forest and back to where we started where we would enjoy another picnic prepared by the convent's kitchen, but no samosas this time. We were shown how the locals would find each other if they got lost in this dense woodland, beating large trunks with branches so that they could be tracked down. And also, the rich reservoirs of water stored in cavities between branches, freshwater always on hand. If you knew your plants you could easily eke out a living, survival, with all the resources that nature offered here.

By the time we got back on the bus it had turned out to be a memorable day, I was really pleased we had made the decision to go with Sheila and that everyone else came along to.

It was a rainforest, but we had been spared the rains. That was until we had got about halfway back to the convent when we had the most torrential rains of our whole fortnight in Kenya. But for all that, it did not spoil our day.

We had a couple more days to finish all that we had wanted to teach and were now ahead of ourselves in where we wanted to be. The rest of the class finished off their presentations to us and did it very well. We were well pleased with what they had produced, and I suppose that was a reflection on what we had tried to get across to them. We had time left before we departed to open the floor to the class to ask anything they wanted, anything they did not understand or anything they quickly wanted us to cover. Then we had the Kenyan director of *Send a Cow* who had arrived to present the class with their certificates of achievement. Well deserved. Lastly, we had a group photo to take, lunch and then Anna and I would be on our way back to Kisumu and a flight back to Nairobi.

In the end we had broken down the barriers between us and them. We had really enjoyed their company and were very moved by the gratitude they showed us for our going over there to teach and to help them. I was really moved and would have to say that it was a real privilege, one of the greatest privileges of my life to have had the opportunity to partake in this project, something I had long wanted to do but with anew found confidence in myself, I had at last achieved. The memories live on.

It was time to get on the bus to say goodbye to everyone as they were off on another field trip, we were waiting for a taxi to take us back to Kisumu airport and then we had a flight to Nairobi. I hoped I would get the chance to meet up with some of them at a later date if I were lucky enough to return to this part of Africa. I hoped sometime in the future that I could go back to see how their work was progressing, how they were reaching out to take more families out of poverty and improve their lives. We will see, I would like to do that but perhaps the charity's emphasis is now changing as other humanitarian problems arise in the countries it works in, refugee camps in Uganda as civil war displaces people in neighbouring countries, always a changing political scene in this area.

Anna and I had been given a few days to have the chance to see a bit more of the country before we flew back to England, four nights before our return flight on the Saturday evening. Our taxi arrived and it was sadly time to wave everyone goodbye for the final time, it was quite emotional for both of us and on our journey back to Kisumu we reflected on what we hoped we had achieved. We had time to kill, and it was a shame we did not divert to the shores of Lake Victoria which were so close to our journey, but we didn't, reaching the airport and then having plenty of time to spend waiting for a plane which did eventually arrive, rather late.

A short flight back to Nairobi made more spectacular by an electric storm lighting up the city as we approached, and then finding our hotel before, late today, our daily downpour arrived.

We had decided that we would like to go on safari and so before we travelled, we had sorted our own arrangements out to take us up to the Aberdare National Park. We would have one night in the Aberdare Country Club before moving onto a hotel,

The Ark, in the game park, overlooking a waterhole where many animals and birds would come to drink. This was close to Treetops where our now late Queen heard of the death of her father, and her accession to the crown.

A comfortable night in the hotel as the skies emptied themselves of rain, then the following morning we headed out of Nairobi on a familiar road to me from my Kenyan visit the following year. Driving through countryside saturated by rains, water eroding the soils of fields and with many of the maize crops looking rather sick from the amount of water they were receiving. It was a far cry seeing all the streams by the side of the roads being torrents, unlike my visit the previous year when every stream was bone dry, the rains had finished six weeks early!

We arrived at the country club, a wonderful old style colonial place with its own golf course. However today, the only occupants of the course were a few giraffes, zebras, and warthog. We had arranged in the afternoon to go on a walking safari in the grounds of the country club, despite the talk of leopards, and headed off in the direction of the nearest waterhole. We saw views of Mount Kenya, my climb the previous year, that was until the skies grew darker and darker, it was that time of day again and we could not be further from cover. We turned back and after a while were pleased to see a jeep coming our way to rescue us. We were grateful to our guide for his time and took ourselves off to our respective lodges, just like a little cottage, for a hot bath and to get into dry clothes. We would meet up later for dinner, first having a drink in the bar, admiring how the deluge was now pouring through the roof above us. Time to find a bucket or two!

Over dinner, Anna told me she had just heard that her grandmother had died but she had decided that she would continue the trip, there was nothing she could do going back early.

We continued our safari as planned, the next day packing our kit before heading off to Solio National Park. This was a chance to see rhino conservation at its best. Solio has been an ongoing project on a one-time farm estate where ethe numbers of black and white rhino have been growing to the extent now that with their successful breeding program, rhinos are now taken from the park to restock other game parks in the country.

We drove to the entrance of the park across sodden tracks, sliding all over the place and waited in anticipation to see these rare animals. We drove and drove and saw nothing, not one animal and were beginning to feel disappointed. But at last, looking towards Mount Kenya again, there was a large herd of buffalo, and soon after that we saw our first rhinos, mainly the white species but there were a few black rhinos. But black rhinos are quite timid, and it was not long before they were disappearing off into the bush in the distance. But at least we had got to see rhinos and so headed off towards a nearby stream and waterhole. There were signs of a recent lion kill, but all we got to see were the remnants of an earlier meal.

It was time to think about heading back towards the hotel, but first going through scrub into open savannah, we came across first a large group of oryx, and then a group of fifty or more white rhinos. An amazing sight, and with such long horns. Our driver stopped and asked if we wanted to get out to look. He was anyway because he wanted a pee behind the jeep.

"Weren't they dangerous?"

"No. Don't worry," our guide said.

We got out and admired these magnificent animals from now more than thirty, forty yards away. If we did not worry them then they would not worry us.

As we stood so close, I said to Anna that I hoped that one day my grandchildren would have the same opportunity that we were now enjoying, that the conservation efforts would continue to be successful and that one of the endangered species could survive for years to come.

One of those sights it was hard to tear yourself away from, but we had to move on, back to the hotel and then onto The Ark for our next stay. It was fascinating just sitting watching the two and froing's of the animals coming to drink, and to consume the salt that the hotel put down for them. Waterbuck, buffaloes, antelope and then emerging from the bush, a pack of hyenas which put the rest of the animals on edge.

The hotel had a warning system, one hoot for an elephant, two for lions, three for leopard. I had gone back out on the veranda overlooking the waterhole for a pre-dinner drink, waiting for Anna to join me, and was already there when the first hoot was sounded. I had already spotted a couple of elephants walking around the waterhole towards the hotel and the salt. We watched these magnificent animals for a while before heading off for food. They were still there when we had eaten before they headed back off into the forest and us to our beds.

The following day we had hired a guide, Silas, to take us into the Aberdares, a drive which would take us most of the day and cover many miles. It was not long before we encountered in thick forest a group of elephants, but we did not loiter for long as one bull did not seem too keen to see us, it was safer to move on. This is a park where they have tried to reintegrate the Bongo, a rare and small antelope, by removing as many of the large predators as they could. We were not fortunate to see one, but again it is a story of the efforts of conservation going on in these game parks.

Our journey was to take us high into the Aberdares, and on the way we would see three waterfalls, Chania, Magura and Karura. Each in turn had their own beauty and individual features. It was fascinating following this what seemed like a small river before it plunged over a rock face to produce such a wonderful view. The paths to the first two, Chania and Magura, were a little treacherous, but having reached the bottom, what a sight to stand in the spray as all this water plunged down the falls, with those strange effects of the light, causing refraction and the waterfall's own rainbows.

Karura was different, not such a powerful fall, but falling a far greater distance down into a rocky gorge. There were several of these small falls here, all dropping further than the eye could see. A wonderful experience and as we got back to the jeep, Silas related to us how in his early days he had come there with a group of tourists only for the jeep to break down. They were stranded and as they sat there with no way form of communication, groups of lions visited them, before wandering off again. They were after thirty-six hours or so, eventually rescued.

We made our way back to The Ark, seeing several deer, antelope, warthog, monkeys and eventually catching up with other groups of elephants, before arriving back for tea.

It was Anna and my last night in Kenya, this time tomorrow we would be waiting at Nairobi Airport for our return flight back to England. It had we reflected been a great trip, worthwhile for our work with *Send a Cow*, and for some of the sights of Kenya we had seen afterwards. The successful conservation projects we had seen, the rains, and all those wonderful and friendly people that had made the trip so worthwhile.

We at last boarded our flight, having gone back to the Country Club first where we enjoyed a fabulous barbeque in the grounds and stopping on the way back to Nairobi to see the Tara River in full flood. It was a wonderful experience, and despite Anna's sad news while we were there, it had been great company. Back at Heathrow, we collected our luggage and then went to meet her husband, her then driving back to the West Country, me boarding a train back to Telford.

A real privilege to go and be involved in the project, and I do stay connected with some of those we taught. It would be appropriate here to thank all my farmers and friends who supported me in my money raising efforts towards the charity with my climb of Mount Kenya the previous year, which enabled me to go on this valuable experience. Also, to Anna for her help and support while we went about our tasks when over there.

As a vet it was a wonderful experience, as a person likewise. I have authored a book about the visit, and more I found of Kenya's peoples and the problems the country faces. It was enlightening to see this project in terms of what of what it is trying to achieve for female empowerment, how hard these women work and how that should be rewarded with a greater say both at home, in their community and in the running of the country.

A most rewarding and enlightening visit. A real privilege.

FOREIGN TRAVEL:

IT MAY HAVE become obvious that I like travelling, especially if it is to Africa. If my choice of activities may have changed from my early days, it has always been nice to get on a ship or plane, or even put the car on a ferry or train and cross the channel, but to be abroad has always been very fulfilling. Those early days of taking the kids, enjoying the sights and the foreign ambience, a couple of days to unwind from the rigors of work before lying back and soaking the sun, working on that suntan that I was so desperate to get.

But of course, it is not only us humans who travel abroad but also a flow of animals to and from Europe and occasionally, even further afield. I think it would be true to say that for myself, and I think I can say for many others then the work involved in this process has always been one of my pet hates.

With the relaxation of Rabies legislation, during my time when I did do some Small Animal work I would have had to deal with a low level of work involving Pet Passports and Rabies vaccination, and from what I recall, that work was never that taxing and was basically ensuring that dogs and cats travelling abroad had received a Rabies jab at the appropriate time before travelling and then blood tested to check that it had worked. There was some sort of certification about worming, sign on the dotted line and Rover was free to go on his holidays with the rest of the family. Whether much has changed over time I could not be sure, it has been a long time since I have had to deal with any of it, or for that matter how much Brexit has changed things. But certainly, as long as all the paperwork is in place then the family pet is free to travel on holiday with their owners. From a family point of view, my sister-in-law's two dogs now resident in Mallorca, travel frequently between the two countries and through France in between. They may even be classed as Spanish citizens, perros, now.

For my part, do I miss it? Definitely not but it never worried me so much as farm livestock travel, which invariably is a one-way journey. In my early days when in Devon, one of our clients participated in the export of young calves to France, presumably to be reared for veal. Whether one believes in the rights or wrongs of the trade, in those days it was going to happen and if one vet in our practice had not signed them off, then someone else would have done so. We did the work though thankfully it ended. The only necessity we needed then was to be accredited as an LVI, a Local Veterinary Inspector, which you needed to be to do such work as Tuberculin testing, Brucellosis testing and to do Anthrax tests. I had an interesting initiation, meeting up with a Ministry man at another farm in Devon to be shown how to do these tests in practice before adjourning to a pub to do some of the theory! Then a repeat in three days to read the TB test we had done and check I was happy in what I was doing, more pub analysis.

We would then have to go and check these calves before they were loaded for their journey over the sea to France. A matter of checking that their ear number matched that on the schedule and making sure that they were all clinically fit to travel, one or two would often get a reprieve if showing any signs of scour or pneumonia. The paperwork was straightforward, ticking off those travelling, deleting those that were not, signing it and they would be ready to go. I personally did not have to do it many times but even in those days, it was a job I never really looked forward to, and one did feel more than a bit sorry for these calves going on this journey from where they would not enjoy a very long life. A brief involvement other than a few Friday afternoons when we would be asked to go and inspect and certify a pile of cattle hides stacked in the corner of a field close to the office, well salted and ready to go somewhere. What could you say other than that was what they were and count how many there were, sign the forms and hope there were no lurking unseen diseases in them. They would be loaded and would be gone. Something where we went through the motions of doing what we had to do but never being happy with it and thankfully I had only to do it on a couple of occasions.

For one reason or another, I cannot remember exactly why but we stopped doing this and I would not be involved in live animal trade again for many years. And it was many years! BSE (Mad Cow Disease) was diagnosed in cattle in the country in the late eighties and because of that the trade in live calves to the continent ceased until 2005/6 when at last the ban was lifted. Somewhere along the line, exporting cattle and sheep was forgotten, certainly in my life and was I worried about that? Not at all! My only involvement would be that occasional Pet Passport which I have described earlier.

It would not be until I arrived in my final practice at Shrewsbury that I would be involved again. By then we had lost our tag as LVIs and were now classed as OVs (Official Veterinarians) and I had a lengthy list of things I was entitled and trained to do from Exports of dogs and cats, farm animals, even equids though I kept quiet about that! Testing as mentioned before, also on the Sheep Scab panel (I had, surprise, surprise, actually received some training for that one), Notifiable Diseases, a long list of about thirteen categories. It would be as an LVI/OV that I would get involved in the 2001 Foot and Mouth outbreak which had such a devastating effect on farming in this country and on my mental (and many others) health.

And so, when I came to my final place of work, I had all these supposed qualifications under my belt, many I hoped that I would never have to use. But I came to a practice that had a diversity of different farmers including many pedigree breeders of sheep and cattle, and some of them had built up a reputation so that when exports were allowed, their animals were highly sort after, mainly as breeding animals to start herds of which ever breed it was in that foreign destination.

Someone would have to be qualified to certify these animals to facilitate the process of exporting and all the paperwork that went with it.

"What panels are you on Rod?" I was asked.

I had to come clean.

"Most of them including export of farm livestock," though I conveniently forgot to mention about equids. So, once again I would be involved in livestock exports, and I would have to admit it has been the one task that I have always hated. Not because of live animal exports as any involvement on my behalf of calves crossing the channel had long gone, but because of the endless and complicated paperwork involved.

As the practice grew, I may have hoped that more of the vets would do some of this work but there seemed a reluctance for them to get involved. The requirements for being allowed to partake in this process were changing, not like in my early days when I was just added to the lists. Now, and I guess it was sensible, you now had to do some training in these procedures online and then pass a test to allow you to be on the panel for exporting livestock. Where it became a bit farcical was that as I had been on the panel for years, I was granted that wonderfully termed phrase, "Grandfather Rights", all that experience I had attained in the past would hold me in good stead for the next four years when I too would have to do this on-line education and test to enable me to continue. That would be the same for TB testing, Anthrax testing, being able to work in Notifiable Disease outbreaks such as Foot and Mouth Disease and towards the end of my career, bird flu (not heard of as a problem in those early days). Others like small animal exports, pet passports, I would let drop and not revalidate as they cropped up. In time I managed to whittle myself down from being on twelve panels down to three when I had retired. But I never managed to lose Livestock exports!

It was good that some of our clients were getting recognised for their breeding of high quality pedigree cattle and sheep, whether they be traditional native breeds or even one or two continental breeds that then recross the channel. That showed how good some of these breeders' reputations had become.

But the paperwork involved I always, as did the other vets, found more than onerous. We were always told about the importance of certification by the Royal College of Veterinary Surgeons, not signing anything we didn't understand or where there is a conflict of interests but we would receive these forms, these Export Certificates from the powers that be (exports would have to be applied for by the breeder), wade our way through the forms then sign them, stamp them with our official OV stamp, copy them and then have a set travelling with the animals, as set retained by the owner and as et retained by us as well as faxing and sending a set to the relevant Government department. That sounds so simple except that the forms were not, with you having to wade through several different paragraphs where you would have to delete a lot of the written word and stamp it, add in various EEC directives about certain diseases, especially guaranteeing them to be TB and Brucellosis free. To do that we had to have official notification from DEFRA to allow us to sign that part.

Some countries or areas of countries had become free of certain diseases such as Infectious Bovine Rhinotracheitis and would obviously want to maintain that status, so again there would be directives putting restrictions on being able to export cattle if they did not meet the disease requirements of those countries that the export was going to.

It would have been nice if these Export Certificates had been simple and just had the necessary information required for that specific export, but they did not hence all the deletions we as the Official Veterinarian had to do. I hated it, especially as we then would have to do all these deletions on a second form written in the language of the country the animals were going to. French I could cope with, but the exports to The Netherlands, to Germany, to Spain and Portugal, and to Romania that I had to deal with, I don't speak a word of their language so one just had to hope that the written word corresponded with that of the English version, and you had deleted the right paragraphs numbered the same as in English. So much for understanding what you were certifying.

I would have to say that sheep were relatively straight forward in that a lot of the exports I had to do were either to the Isle of Man or to Ireland, so of course the only language I was dealing with was my own. The few times that I had to send sheep across the channel, they were usually going to a holding centre somewhere so it would be the vet there who would eventually have to deal with the export certification, all I would have to do is to do any relevant blood testing for certain diseases, and sign them off as being free when the results arrived back. The sheep then with my inspection that they were healthy within twenty-four hours of them leaving the farm, were permitted to go on to the holding centre and the hassles would be passed on to someone else.

This rarely happened with cattle that I was involved with in exporting, with them invariably leaving the farm direct to a port where they would stay loaded on their transport until they reached their destination the other side. They would be required to have official rest periods for feed and water along the way for what would be a long journey, but the lorry drivers were experienced at their work and would look after all the welfare requirements of the cattle.

Over my time, I found that other of the vets would not revalidate their export panel and so it became increasingly likely that this work would always fall on one other vet and myself, more often than not, me!

It would be a requirement that the cattle would have to be Tuberculin tested within thirty days of travelling, this sometimes causing an issue if for some reason the transport, the shipment was delayed. If this happened and they fell outside this period, then another test could not take place for sixty days after this test. One found oneself almost having to manage the shipment oneself to make sure it would happen, and as I have said before, this was far from my favourite job, in fact I hated it.

So, I guess an explanation to why my feelings on this particular part of our work (and for those who gave up or did not want to do it) is due. It was basically the paperwork which as I have said before is more than complicated with adding the right directives, deleting the right parts and some of the statements are more than a bit ambiguous. I never knew why in granting the export certificate why Animal Health offices (as they are now) could not produce a bespoke certificate for each export because the basic needs of one country would always be the same. It seemed to me that they just complicated the procedure with this one certificate fits all, just cross out the bits you think do not apply.

I would do the Tuberculin test and if all were clear we would get the process underway, hoping that the relevant certificate would be faxed in time to print off. Then within twenty-four hours of the departure of the cattle from the farm, I would visit the farm and inspect the cattle to be sure there were no signs of disease, they were fit and healthy to travel. All being well, I would then have to complete the form (I may have already filled in some of it before arriving on the farm. Then providing the farmer would have a photocopier, when it was all signed, stamped in the appropriate way and in the right places (they liked the papers fanned out to stamp so your official stamp would cover every sheet), it would be copied in triplicate with all necessary papers clipped together to be distributed to those that needed a copy, the originals travelling with the animals.

Straight forward, should be, but with the complicated forms I and many others would worry until we had heard that they had arrived safely at their destination and probably for a couple of days after that, waiting to be sure that the paperwork had been filled in properly. At least on reaching their destination one knew that the port authorities had accepted it, but the central authorities could often be very pedantic.

For Bob I assisted in the export of many cattle, especially heifers and a few adult cows to Holland. I had met the farmer from over there who was the buyer and so with his forms, one got accustomed to the paperwork involved. At one stage, when Blue Tongue had raised its ugly head as a new disease in this country, a virus transmitted by a certain type of midge, cattle had to be vaccinated before travel as well as treated with an insecticide prior to loading. This too had to be certified that it had been carried out. The Blue Tongue vaccine required two injections and if both were given on the same farm, I could sign for both. But on one occasion, the heifer, which was going to Northern Ireland, had been given her first jab on another farm in Cheshire by another vet. That meant that she needed two certificates of vaccination, one from him and one from me who administered the second.

I had collected all the relevant paperwork together, including the export certificate and as it was all in my language, thought everything should be simple.

I think over time that I found out that anything going to Northern Ireland was more complicated than for anywhere else. The heifer went complete with all her paperwork, I had checked it all several times and of course had my own copies. She would go up to Liverpool, onto the ferry and over to Larne to be unloaded and then delivered to her new owners, that simple, and off she went with as far as I was concerned, no complications.

Later that night I had a call from the port authorities at Larne. The certificate of first vaccination was not there, and without it they would have to put her on the next ship back. The officer said he could not allow her off the boat without this and I should have been more careful with my paperwork.

This was exactly why I hated exports!

I knew it was there and asked him to go through all the documents once again, he would find it. He checked again but to no avail, he would have to send the heifer back without unloading her. Once again, I asked him to recheck all the papers, I knew I had sent it and could not see why one sheet had gone missing. "No," he informed me, "It wasn't there."

I was getting a little distraught and anxious because I was so certain it had gone with the rest of the documents, though now being at home I did not have my copies with me. I asked him to look again to no avail, and then one last time I went through each document he should have and where this certificate should be.

It was no surprise to me that at last he found it, though did I get an apology or anything? No, I did not for what had been more than a few minutes of him causing me more than a little distress. I was more than relieved he had found it and that the heifer could be unloaded in Ireland and complete her journey, but had it increased my love of exporting, definitely not.

It was time for me to revalidate and did I really want to for one last time as this next period would take me to after my planned retirement date. I did not really want to but we who could do it were thin on the ground by now, so I was persuaded to carry on. By now, the revalidation course had taken on epic proportions with me having to learn about equid requirements for Europe, as well as such common day to day tasks as to what I needed to know if I had to deal with the likes of elephants. And with my multiple-choice test that I had to pass at the end of the course, was there in it of much relevance to cattle and sheep. Certainly not, deer, horses, pachyderms. Yes, but little of the stock I dealt with.

So, I continued this unenviable task until near retirement, a few sheep as before and mainly for Bob with his pedigree sales to the continent. I did have to certify a group of Jersey cattle going to a far warmer climate, Saudi Arabis who were trying to develop their own milk industry, and some cattle to Spain. Otherwise, it was much as it had been, and with one of the younger vets taking on some of the sheep exports life got a little easier on this side for me. I would have to give him advice now and again from my experiences in the past, but I did not mind doing that.

Otherwise, the other main pain was one farmer who more than once would ring on a Sunday when I was on call, I think it may have happened when I was not on call as well. He would ring to say that he had a lorry or jeep and trailer coming within the hour to pick up a young bull or valuable heifer and he needed the export certificate for her signing. This would put a great strain on me, firstly because if I was on call this was time consuming and suppose an urgent call came in, a real emergency. Secondly, I knew nothing about the export, nor did the practice so where was all the necessary paperwork. One would have to track that down, complete it, get it all, signed up and stamped while an impatient driver waited, wanting to leave as soon as possible so he could travel upto Stranraer to get the ferry to go over to Ireland. The only good thing was that it was only up the road from the office so getting all the photocopying done to get the duplicates of the forms was easy. But it was always a real pain to do this at short notice and of course it was always our fault that we knew nothing about it.

I do not know how we did it sometimes, but the cattle did always get away but because it had been so rushed, I worried for ages expecting that phone call that I had done something wrong. Plus, the Irish lorry driver would always produce another form which he said needed to be signed for cattle to get into Ireland, the most important piece of paper of them all. I often thought did I have the authority to sign it, and if it was so important, then why did it not come with the proper export papers.

I did get a couple of phone calls from the powers that be about paperwork over my time, sometimes helpful and advisory, on one occasion a bit stroppy and on that occasion did beg the question of why the forms had to be so complicated and why couldn't they just be presented relevant to that particular export so we wouldn't have to delete half the form. I did not get a satisfactory answer!

Over my last couple of years, with Brexit and the official leaving of the EEC, the export trade dried up. Troubles with Border Controls made it difficult to get animals out of the country. I cannot say I was that sorry and when I was asked when I retired if I was happy to continue doing the odd export if required, my answer was a firm no. Not long after, my revalidation would come up again and there was no way I was going to take the course again.

Thankfully and much to my relief, my days of exporting cattle and sheep were well and truly over. Boy, was I glad.

Easily the part of my career I least liked and do not miss it at all. Bob still gets enquires from the Netherlands, but it is still not easy to get his cattle over the North Sea. One thing is for certain though, it will not be me doing the paperwork and signing them off, that task will fall on some other lucky (or not so lucky) soul.

THE PEDIGREE
BREEDER:

CHANGING TIMES HAVE meant changes in the needs of farmers and with that some change in what we must do in the veterinary profession to serve them. Management changes, better feeding regimes, the course of time looking for more and better ways of producing the feed to put on our tables. With that has been the wish to improve the breeding stock that we have, improving the genetic potential so that certain traits can be bred for, increased milk yield, better feed conversion, improved live weight gain and better carcase quality would be naming just a few. The science that goes into selecting these traits and how they are measured are beyond me but as well as having the advantage of using sexed semen to use on your better cows to guarantee (almost) that you will have a heifer calf from these cows, one can select different sires to improve certain traits from each individual animal. The complete breeding program! This means that those animals that you do not want to keep in terms of genetic merit can be bred to beef bulls. Of course, there is the same amount of genetic selection that can go into the breeding of these bulls.

This is where our pedigree breeders have their role, producing the breeding stock to use both on our beef suckler herds and to produce cross-bred calves to sell off dairy farms onto fattening units to produce the beef that goes on to your tables. Those similar traits will be looked for in both the sheep and the pig industries as well. Genetic monitoring and selection have become increasingly important.

The export industry which I have just described will be to

improve the breeding stock in their intended destinations, and likewise a flow of cattle into this country especially from Holland to go into our dairy herds. It seems a shame that even some of our traditional breeds such as David's Jerseys, then now even some of them are sourced from foreign shores and not from our own herds in this country.

The pedigree breeder, and I have been lucky enough to be involved with a few of them! That has been an involvement in pedigree sheep, in dairy cattle and in some of our beef breeds. That involvement in dairy cows has been with farmers wanting to improve their own stock although along the way they may rear on a bull calf which potentially has high genetic merit and can be sold on to another farmer to improve his progeny. To be honest, if there has been anything I have dealt with in these cases, it has usually been to evaluate that they are specific disease free, to ensure especially some of the viral diseases affecting our national herd are not passed on to the next farm. Highly infectious diseases that can severely affect the fertility and general health in a naïve herd, so we are trying to offer a safety net in controlling the spread of these diseases. IBR and BVD have been mentioned several times in my previous writings, diseases where in certain countries there is an eradication plan and hopefully one day, we in England may obtain that free status. We are more than a little way off with that now, relying more on a vaccination policy, but one day that will change for the long-term benefit of the national herd.

Sheep again there has been some involvement which I have undertaken but that has been more with general flock health and involvement in export of pedigree rams. Again, there has been some blood testing against certain diseases but most work has been what I would do with most commercial flocks except that these are pedigree and so far, more valuable. It is staggering the amount some of these sheep change hands for, rams often being far more expensive than a pedigree bull to tidy up your calving pattern or to use to run with heifers.

But the beef breed side of the pedigree industry has been more interesting with different requirements on the different farms I have worked with. When I started in practice there was a change from the traditional British beef breeds such as the Hereford and the Aberdeen Angus to some of the larger Continental breeds such as the Charolais and the Limousin. Belgian Blues came over with their vast hind leg muscling, Simmentals were popular for a while, the Blonde Aquitaine was another, each being in fad for a time but then losing their popularity. How many calvings would I have done especially in my early days when one of these breeds, especially the Charolais, would be the sire and you put your hand inside a heifer to feel this massive pair of feet and you knew from the onset that it would not come out of the right passageway. Another caesarean and one hoped that the farmer had not damaged the animal too much in his efforts to calve her before calling the vet out. Over time, education taught the farmer that a small live calf and a healthy heifer was far more valuable than a damaged heifer and a dead calf. Sometimes one would be rewarded (if that is the right word) with a massive live calf which would top the market when sent there, but the risk was not worth taking.

We went back to smaller breeds of bulls thankfully, though even some of those breeds now get larger. The Hereford once known for its easy calving traits, perhaps now has got large in the shoulder and they are not so easy to calve now.

But what of some of my breeders and my involvement?

Bob started his business in the meat trade and had done very well out of it so that he was able to buy a house with a small acreage attached to it. What should he do with it other than getting an expensive lawn mower to cut the grass frequently. He decided to get a few cattle to keep it grazed down and at the end of their cycle he would have something to sell into his first trade, meat. His introduction into the life of a farmer was with a few Simmental cattle.

But that small introduction into the cattle world had sparked an interest as well as saving him having to cut the grass. From his background in his main job, he knew what he required in a beef animal and to that end he developed an interest in the Angus breed, not so much the traditional Scottish Aberdeen Angus but the larger Canadian Angus type. When those first few cattle had gone, Bob soon took himself up to the Angus breed sales in Carlisle and before long he had the start of his own Angus herd. This slowly grew as he became more interested in breeding his own cattle and before long as this interest grew, he had outgrown his small holding and needed a bigger farm.

A farm outside Newport became available which Bob purchased and that was the start of the Penguin herd of Angus cattle at Windy Meadows. Over the following years, Bob's interest in the breed grew and grew and as he expanded the size of his herd, he found that this new "hobby" was benefitting him in other ways. He got himself involved with the breed society and through that he met new people, fellow breeders of Angus cattle so he obtained new friendships, more social interaction with his new comrades and was able to involve both himself and his wife in this new interest.

As time progressed, he built up his own reputation amongst the breeders, becoming increasingly involved in the breed society, eventually reaching to be the top man, president for a year and being on its committee. Being invited to judge the breed at shows would soon follow, as well as selling pedigree bulls at society shows and topping the market. His cattle were now highly sought after both as breeding bulls and for selling heifers for other breeders to develop their own herd. The exports that I have already mentioned were proof of his esteemed name in the breed society.

He would become a frequent visitor to Canada to see some of the top breeding animals over there and to purchase embryos to bring back to this country to improve his own genetics in the herd.

He had from those small beginnings become a breeder of some renown and an important person in the breed society.

Of course over time, age catches up with us all and with no-one else in the family to continue his work, he reached a time when it was time to downsize considerably, it was time to sell most of the herd while keeping a few cattle to maintain his own interest as well as giving him something of a small hobby in later life.

For me, I have been attending his cattle throughout my career in Shropshire. There may have been times when I have moved practice or he has changed his vets for personal treasons but we always throughout my career in Shropshire have become interlinked, I have always ended up being his vet wherever I have worked, and that interest has continued past my retirement date.

It has been interesting doing his work for him, partly through the array of cases I have had to deal with but also because of the other people I have worked with while on his farm. Fraser, a keen Angus man himself, who thought he knew everything but probably did not, but was a particularly good stockman who knew how to handle cattle and get them ready for shows and sales. There is a skill in training a young bull, full of himself, but who needed to be halter broken and be easy to manage. When fully grown, these bulls are big chaps but needed to be taught to respect humans.

People like Bob (another Bob) who I had worked with on a couple of different farms before here, and Pete, good conscientious stockmen, especially in Bob's case as he was brilliant at getting calves going in their early life, having the patience to milk a stroppy mother not used to hand milking so that he could feed her calf with her own milk. Some of these cows either had such low udders that the calf did not know how to access the milk, or she was just reluctant to let the calf suck to begin with and had to be trained to let it.

There was another who thought he knew everything until he managed to half demolish one of the sheds with the fore loader on the tractor, spectacular but not helpful. And he seemed to book himself off on holiday for most of the summer, not an immense help.

But all of them I got on well with and was always glad of their assistance for the times I was called to visit. And their help was appreciated.

He had started his herd from nothing, built it up for him to be a top breeder in his chosen breed. All things end at some stage, we all cannot go on forever and at the end of my career, it was also time for Bob to call an end to his. A herd dispersal sale would be the end of the herd, the end of a lifetimes work. But he will retain a few cattle, which will give him some interest in his later years, and with the herd under a new prefix.

Farming not that far away from Bob, Christine first showed an interest in cattle when her father bought a small holding back in 1980 and acquired a few commercial cattle, Limousin cross South Devons, to fatten, and then a few suckler cows to bred from and start his own herd. Christine soon developed an interest herself and before long between them they had acquired a larger premises and their stock numbers had gone up appreciably. A hundred and fifty cattle, different breeds ranging from the British Hereford to imported Charolais' and more exotic Italian breeds. You name the breed, and they were on the farm! An interest in both the commercial and showing side of cattle breeding was starting to develop. By 1989 Christine was concentrating her efforts into fewer breeds, now starting to specialise in her Limousins and a couple of other continental breeds, specifically now for breeding top quality pedigree animals to go to other breeding herds, for showing and for selling the not quite so good bulls to for commercial use as stock bulls on suckler and dairy farms. The Wilodge name had started and was gaining a reputation for the cattle that it was producing.

Over the years, she continued with her commitment to producing top quality beef breeding animals and was joined by her now husband Paul. He not only had an interest in the cattle but also in sheep, having started a small flock in his native Somerset in the late eighties, and then expanding the enterprise in breeding Texels to begin with, but then Beltex, Blue Texels and Border Leicester sheep. He also had a commercial flock, producing lamb for our butcher markets.

Between Paul and Christine, they were exploring how to maximise the potential of their top-quality breeding stock. Like a lot of pedigree breeders, they investigated how they could increase the potential of their best breeding families, how to multiply those families quickly, both in the sheep and the cattle. Technology was improving on the side of embryo transfer so by flushing their best breeding cows to super ovulate them, producing multiple eggs at one bulling, they could then harvest these embryos and implant them into other breeding cattle when needed. Our role as vets in this was to check the cows were in prime condition for breeding, their ovaries were functioning normally, and to synchronise a group of usually heifers to come bulling at the same time so that when the specialised technicians who did the embryo transfers wanted to proceed, the recipients of these fertilised eggs could all be implanted at the same time. A slightly different technique with the sheep, but again multiple fertilised eggs could be harvested from the best pedigree ewes and implanted in commercial sheep to produce high genetic merit lambs.

The system worked very well, achieving satisfactory results and for us as the vets, it worked well in that we knew when calvings/ lambings were expected (concentrated in an abbreviated period of time as they were synchronised together). We could be ready and prepared for their requirements of us at their calving/ lambing times. It was a system that functioned well with periods of when breeding took place, but spacing this over several time intervals so that one group could be supervised and receive top quality management, and when this group was established and healthy, the next group could then receive the same treatment.

I enjoyed helping to work in this system, also doing pregnancy diagnosis sessions to confirm that those cows that had an embryo implanted in them had retained the pregnancy, and of course there would be the obstetrical work at the end of the cycle.

The rewards, the best animals, young bulls and heifers, and likewise young rams and ewes would goi to the big pedigree sales in the autumn months, especially at Carlisle but also with the sheep along the borders with Wales. There would be the big shows, the Highland, Royal Welsh for example, where the top animals would go into the ring to be judged against other breeders' top stock with much success being a reward for Christine and Paul's breeding policies. With success, you get asked to be a judge yourself, as did Bob, and especially Paul now performs those duties at breed shows.

The top-quality animals would be sold to other pedigree herds and flocks, the not so good ones to commercial herds and those that were classed as not good enough would be fattened for beef and lamb. There was a structure in this breeding policy serving several sectors of meat production.

Talking about the economics of it all is interesting and Paul would explain to me that the end product has not really gone up in price over the last few years, but the costs have. To produce a bull or heifer for sale as a breeding animal one is looking at selling them at eighteen months old where a bull is ready to be used as a sire, heifers ready to get in calf. With a nine-month gestation period, Paul explained that you are looking at twenty-seven months plus to get a return on your investment. But costs have gone up, feed, fertilizer, as it has for all farmers. But then there are the registration costs for the breed, DNA testing, plus the costs of flushing, embryo transfer and more as technology progresses, which have not got any cheaper, the margins have got less. With the sheep there is a far quicker return on the capital outlay, with a five-month gestation period and then if you wanted, you could breed from the progeny that year. Paul explained to me, which I had often wondered why, that was the reason that tups made more money at the pedigree sales than bulls do.

A top-quality Limousin is a beautiful animal to look at, prime beef on the hoof. Perhaps now though Paul and Christine have looked at other ways to produce cattle, another market, the top fatstock sales and especially those Christmas markets where silly money exchanges hands for the prestige of buying the best animal at the market. The number of Limousins on the farm has been reduced to the top families so that now there are only a dozen pedigrees left, but here are plenty of embryos frozen in storage for future use. British Blue bulls are used on some of the breeding animals to produce big, muscled beef animals for these fatstock sales, and it is now the case that one of these bulls will make as much money if not more that an average breeding bull. Dairy farmers do not seem to want to spend a lot of money on a bull, and the national suckler herd is diminishing as increased numbers of beef calves now come from dairy herds. With the use of sexed semen, it has streamlined a dairy farmer breeding system so that they can serve more cows to beef as they can target their best dairy cows to serve with dairy bulls, being more than certain they will get a heifer calf.

It has been fun helping Christine and Paul try and achieve their aims, even the middle of the night calvings and lambings. Working for them has always been good humoured with facilities that made my job easier.

And the ultimate reward for them, getting the top price for a heifer in a pedigree sale, a record, for Posh Spice, a couple of years ago. Her progeny will soon be available on the market, and it will be interesting to see the sort of money they make.

And who knows, one day Paul and Christine may produce another valuable heifer like her, a reward for their hard work and their selective breeding policies. Technology moves on, IVF in cattle and sheep. Where will the future take us with these developments, only time will tell but at the moment, Wilodge will continue to be at the forefront of producing the best pedigree animals of their breeds.

For me, I will view their success from a distance, staying connected with them but continuing to show an interest in what these now good friends are trying to achieve.

And with Bob with his Angus's, again I am keen to see where he goes from here with his small herd which I do still have a little involvement with.

At the end of the day, I enjoy a good steak and that is what it is all about.

Retirement and Reflection:

I T WAS TIME to start a new life. My working days were now over, and it was now all "my" time, the chance to do all those things that I had always wanted to do but never had the time. I had discovered myself late in my life, which is late in my life so far and there was so much more I wanted to do, health and finances allowing. There was even the occasional talk of going back to Africa and trying Kilimanjaro again or perhaps Mount Kenya and reaching the top. Those thoughts Jane had banned, but a man has to do what a man has to do to reach his destiny. Watch this space!

Jane always moaned that I never had any hobbies, but am I a man who can never sit still? That is me. How many times had I played golf over the past few years, and with Covid our regular meet ups with the boys to watch England rugby internationals and play did not happen, the fairways of England awaited my presence. Walking, climbing, and enjoying nature, the wonderful British countryside were all on the agenda. My annual trip up to the Lakes would happen again, and even before retirement had set in, a phone call from a hotel Jane and I had visited a couple of years previously had offered a special deal on a short break which we were only to keen to accept. The only question would be was when we could fit it into our schedule, it looked like it would have to be April 2022, nearly a year after I had finished. That may have partly been governed by making sure we were not in the mosquito season, it is me they seem to like eating, not Jane!

So, in the beginning of June 2021 my new life began with a few days in Bala and then an extended stay in Symmondsbury, Dorset. I would have to say this new lifestyle really suited staying in a quiet village, blending into rural life. The village pub, meeting new people, regular hikes up Colmer Hill to watch the sunset over the Jurassic coast and of course one of our favourite places, the beach and pub at Seatown though with Covid restrictions there, getting a beer was often a challenge. The beach bar and just enjoying a pint of Dorset Gold over a barbeque while watching the ebbing and flowing of a gentle tide was more than relaxing and just the life for me. My son came down for a couple of nights and it was great to spend some real time with him; father and son though more now, just two very good friends just chatting away. Golf with Graham and Anthony at Axe Cliff, yes that return to a sport that had left me behind, but alas with a few old duffers in front of us, progress was so slow that we gave up after eleven holes, if we had followed them much longer the next ice age may have started.

It was a wonderful break and showed me the type of life I wanted to lead now my working career was finished, and where I wanted to lead that life, but alas, Dorset was financially way out of Jane and my reach.

I also knew that despite my retirement, I still had the odd job or two to do veterinary wise, and I had told my old job that if they were short-handed then I would do some TB testing for them. Tuberculosis in cattle was still rife in our part of Shropshire, and with many farms requiring testing every sixty days it was highly likely that at some stage my services would be called upon.

So, I did have some sort of plan to work to, and a sort of a figure I had in my head of what money I needed to earn in my first year of non-work, especially if Jane was not going to work.

June was a glorious month of wind down, relax and think of the future and where it would take me. A great summer to get into the practice of this retirement game, but I didn't want to lose contact with some of those farmers who had become firm friends, even more so because with Covid restrictions I had not seen them as much as I had wanted over my final few days, weeks as a vet.

July saw me returning to TB testing, just one herd helping a friend out. A test that I had done many times in the past but now, probably for the last time. I think the previous time I had done this particular farm; I had said that was the last time. But when asked, though this was a slow and sometimes frustrating test to do, I was extremely happy to help out. A sunny day and working with cattle, it had been my whole life, then I would do it. All went well and it was a little bit of pocket money to see me through the summer.

I did do the odd jobs for other people privately, nothing too strenuous and only things within my limitations of what equipment I still possessed and where it fitted into my "retirement" diary. I was finding out what a pleasure it was to oversee my own time, no early starts, no late finishes and no out of hours. And it was good to keep my hand in calving the odd cow or two, I still had it in me.

My life was my own! I had now been asked if I could do some TB testing but that would be in late September through to mid-November, working four days a week, Monday, Tuesday, Thursday and Friday, the days as long as the tests took me. But that eight-week period also included a trip to Mallorca for a few days and a long weekend in Bristol for my son's stag do.

But first we, Jane and I, would take ourselves off to Llandudno to have a look at the place if this is where we thought was the place to which we would retire. A journey that would take us through Flint then along the coast, Rhyl, Prestatyn, Conway and Rhos-on-Sea before dropping down into Llandudno to stay at a delightful Airbnb in a quiet part of town close to the seafront. We had delightful hosts who were only too keen to act as a taxi service for us in the evening so we could have a drink or two in Snoozes, an excellent restaurant, without having to worry about the car. Exploring the Great Orme, using the tram to climb up and meeting interesting people while on the tram, admiring the views towards Snowdonia and over to Anglesey. There were crowds but then people were holidaying in Britain rather than foreign travel because of the Covid vaccinations and documentation you needed to travel abroad.

Jane took the tram down, queuing to get on it, I arranged to meet her at the end of the pier as I was going to walk down, but I beat her by minutes, several, and so walked up to the tram stop.

A bus tour of the area the next day, getting off and on when we wanted to would give us a further look at the area and any possible locations we may want to settle. Then it was time to return home, again along the coast, stopping for Jane to look at a fabric outlet store (her hobby, embroidery and we had found a nice shop in Llandudno for her) while I took a lovely walk along the Dee estuary coast path, a great walk and something I wasn't expecting, such great scenery.

September would see us back in Llandudno, VIPs at the Tour of Britain cycle race, and again what a wonderful day, something I would never have envisaged in my working days spending a day watching cycling. We were on the finish line, again at the top of the Great Orme and after being wined and dined graciously, we couldn't have expected a more exciting finish than the best two cyclists in the race Wout Van Aert and Julian Alaphillippe after two hundred mountainous kilometres of racing, being separated on the finish line by half a backside. Memorable.

But it was time to think about being a vet again, although only very briefly, the six-week period I had said I would do spanning over eight weeks. I needed to be logged back into the system for submitting tests online, like everything else TB testing was now becoming more technical. There was even a cow side machine now that you could record the cow's ear number and her skin thickness readings while you were doing the test, then electronically transferring all this information onto a computer you were logged in on, instant submission of the test. But for my little non-technological b rain that was too much, I was quite happy to submit tests the way I had for many years now. I just needed to be able to log on to the system, and Siobhan with her normal efficiency made all that possible along with supplying me with the necessary equipment and disinfectants I would need to perform my duties for those few weeks.

I had spent over three months away from a working environment, and it would be interesting to see how I would adapt back to it although only briefly. I had had time to reflect on a new life away from work, and I would have to say that I was thoroughly enjoying it other than missing farming and its contacts, it had been my whole life up to this point. As a lot of people say on retirement, "how did I ever find time for work?" My time was being occupied fully. Maybe there was even a little resentment in my mind of the things that I would have to put on hold while I spent these next few weeks working. I would also reflect on how much more intimate I had become with nature especially with my walking, spending far more time watching the bird life around, the flowers, the different barks on trees and observing how less timid the likes of squirrels had become. Was that because of Covid and furlough that many more people were walking and cycling, using the facilities the town park in Telford offered for outdoor pursuits.

All that was on hold for the time being as I donned my wellies again for work. My first week back was a gentle introduction. Day one was a lunchtime start with a suckler herd in the middle of nowhere but with a farmer I knew, a test I have described earlier. A hundred odd Longhorns to test, trying to avoid the points of their extraordinarily long horns as they swung their heads back and forth. I arrived at the map reference destination, now in my nearly new Qashqai. Somewhere along the line we, Jane and I, had decided not to use it for work or off-roading. I had at last sold my last trusty Vauxhall Vectra a few weeks previously so had no option but to use this car for work now. And here I was in front of a gate with a track extending forwards up and over a hill, into the distance. So much for plans, I headed up across the field in my new car, at last finding a cattle crush, the cattle and part of the farm team waiting amongst an oak wood, this was very rural parkland grazing with plenty of falling acorns and old branches lying about. But then, the final product from this farm was traditional organic beef, the setting was very apt.

While I was doing the Tb test, I had also been asked to blood test the breeding herd for three diseases, and depending on the results if we had them in time, the farmer would vaccinate the herd against Bovine Viral diarrhoea and Bovine Infectious Rhinotracheitis when I read the test three days later. The third test, for Neospora would suggest whether any positive testing cows should be retained for breeding as the disease invariably causes abortion, or if the calf does survive, it will usually be positive as well. We wanted to try and eradicate it from the herd. It is a disease caused by an organism, the adult part of its life cycle being in dogs and foxes who then excreted the infective part of their lifecycle in their faeces. If picked up by cattle who are the hosts of the next part of their life cycle, this is where the problems in reproduction take place. It is important that dogs are kept under control on these grazing lands and that their faeces are collected and disposed of in an appropriate way.

But I digress, what was a nice sunny day when we started turned into an absolute deluge which continued with the rain continuing to drip off the leaves of these magnificent oaks. Testing, I got wet, but doing the paperwork as we went along was becoming more challenging the wetter we and it got. The joys of being a vet!

But eventually we did finish, and I would have to get all the paperwork for the blood tests completed and sent off before I started my next test the following day. This was duly done before I set off for my days' work, to test two cows on one farm. They had tested inconclusive sixty days previously; I was to decide their fate and what future testing regime the farmer would continue with. An easy day's work but for me a waste of a day as I had so little to do.

The end of the week saw me reading these tests. The Longhorns, we had received the results of the blood tests and were able to go ahead vaccinating, it soon becoming obvious that it was easier for me to be doing this as well as reading the Tb test, while the others got the cattle into the race. There were some positive to Neospora infection, these would be culled out. A clear test for Tb much to the relief of the farmer, I would submit it the following morning before going to my brief test of two cattle. This thankfully was also clear, the cows could return to the herd but there would always be a worry over them, two inconclusive tests turn into a reactor!

A short day, but I had a train to catch. It was my son's stag do in Bristol. The best man had managed to secure enough accommodation in a Travelodge near the Docks, but it meant us having to share rooms.

I travelled down by train, Jane dropping me off at Telford Central. I would change at Birmingham New Street to take me to Bristol Templemeads (an old familiar name from my student days) then I would walk the mile and a bit to the hotel, hoping to arrive by mid-afternoon when the "action" was due to begin. It was nice travelling through the countryside of Worcestershire and Gloucestershire before arriving in the city I had spent my student days.

A What's App group had been set up so people could give their progress from various parts of the country and their expected arrival time. I was not going to be the first, definitely not the last. I walked to the hotel and sent a message of my arrival. The stags had already departed to the first pub on the list. As I was checking in, the next guest arrived, my daughter's fiancée, also from Telford. We had travelled down on the same busy train, and it was only now that we had bumped into each other. I found my room; I was alone for the night and would not have to worry about any snoring disturbing a roommate.

We found out where the stag party was and set off along the docklands to find them, they were on their way to pub number two. Hopefully someone knew the way, we did eventually find it where we waited until the rest of the party joined us. Over the years I had met several of Richard's university and work colleagues, all now a little older but great to catch up with them, a friendly bunch. Others, I had not met before, but it soon became obvious that most people were called Matt, and if not then were Tom's. It was great to meet all these good friends of my son, plus one or two others who had come for this evening as there were one or two spare tickets, we were going to see Bristol play Bath, a local derby, at rugby.

On to Ashton Gate, someone managed to get hold of some beer, and then the walk back through the docks to the City Centre. What a vibrant place Bristol was now compared with my student days, despite the Covid worries still, no end of people sitting at wooden benches outside pubs and enjoying the ambiance of a mild early autumn evening. More beer but now approaching midnight, I really thought food would be good. We found a food bar eventually, but I would have to admit that my "KFC" equivalent was disgusting and ended up in the nearest bin. On an empty stomach and needing a loo I thought it time to retire for the evening back to the hotel and let the youngsters continue as they seemed fit. I gather it was Richard's idea to go to a club where they continued until gone four in the morning.

They were playing football at ten the next morning, I was not!

I rose to find one or two of the others trying to find some breakfast nearby. I walked to the local Tesco Express to buy a paper and a bacon sandwich in what I remember as typical Bristol weather, it was raining! When back at the hotel, everyone was getting ready to go to the other side of Bristol to play football, my morning was planned with a trip around S.S Great Britain, something I would recommend to anyone visiting the city. And my ticket gave me entry for the following twelve months, I hoped I would get the chance to use it again.

After finding a nice café near the waterfront and enjoying a rather scrummy avocado baguette I returned to the hotel to find everyone else now returned but in much confusion, rooms had been swapped around by the management, keys no longer worked, and it took a considerable time to sort it all out.

We had to be back in the city centre to play darts in a new complex where you hired an ockey, were served food and drinks if wanted and your score, order of throwing etc was all done electronically, shown up in front of you. Next was more beer, we had about four hours to kill before our table at an Indian was available. My son was starting to look a little worse for wear, where was the best man to look after him? It was left for dad to help the lad out; fresh air and a spell of non-alcoholic beverage was the order of the day. I did meet the person I was to spend that night with, he had arrived late to the stag do because of family commitments and assured me he could sleep through anything. Chris, I think, I had met some years earlier when Richard shared a flat with him in Brixton. I had used his bed then until he returned from a weekend away.

The rest of the evening passed peacefully, Richard sticking with the elderly fraternity and finding nowhere else staying open late, returned to the hotel for a night cap and earlier night. Others went to a night club, my roommate included. I took his things to our room and hoped he would not disturb me when he came in. In the morning, he was dead to the world and rather than disturbing him, I took myself back to Templemeads to catch the first available train back to Birmingham and then Telford. Bristol was dead at that time on a wet Sunday morning, even the station where I had to wait for an hour to catch the train. I think other than our introduction, those were the only words said between Chris and I until the wedding day, where at the reception I was seated near him, Jane between us. I did pass the comment that perhaps I should be in the middle, with the only two people I had slept with that year either side of me!

A lovely weekend being able to share time and space with Richard and his friends, and to reflect on how much Bristol had changed since my student days.

It was time to go back to work, and the Monday morning would be an easy start, but a test where patience would be a virtue, not a real problem in my chilled state. Testing at a small family farm, a hundred and fifty odd animals and a chance to renew old acquaintances, a chat over a cup of coffee and then on to do two small tests.

My last test of the day at Stonehaven took me back to a small holding I had visited just over three years previously when I had done his first test of one heifer. He had a few sheep and poultry, but this was only going to be a hobby. But he was then extremely interested in my shortly coming up trip to Kenya with *Send a Cow*, and on seeing him again he was keen to learn my experiences when out there. For something that had been such a privilege to do, it was a pleasure to pass on details of the wonderful work that the charity is doing in East Africa.

Perhaps the next day was the one that I had been dreading, having to do an early start again, the first for a long time and certainly the first in retirement, getting up at four to be on farm by five. I had not lost the ability of not sleeping for an early, just lying there waiting for the alarm to go off. I just hoped the lighting would be good enough to be working in the dark, especially when arriving on the farm which seemed deserted. The cowman arrived soon after, then my helpers. It was an efficient test before being offered a cooked breakfast, was I going to say no? Here was a chance to talk about the changing farming scene, something I really enjoyed.

We had to go to two more farms to finish the test, the only problem being one missing heifer. We searched the fields high and low for her, but she was absent without leave. The farmer did go back later in the day and did find her escaped into another field, but it did mean that going back later, the test was completed all on the same day.

Week three of testing and two big tests but not starting at atrociously early hours of the morning, two farms on restrictions as they had previous Tb reactors, and for the first time in my career I was going to have to test goats as well. But two very enjoyable tests, efficient and a pleasure to work in the company of such nice farmers. The first, when we finished, offered me a cup of coffee. I commented that did they want to fail when my coffee arrived in a Liverpool FC mug, I informed them I was a United fan! The test the next day with Pete and Colin, we knew each other as United fans and here was a chance to put the world right with the present travails of the club.

It was an enjoyable week of testing in what was lovely October weather.

Week four of testing would be curtailed by Jane and I flying off to Mallorca for an enjoyable break with her sister, walking, relaxing, helping on the finca and enjoying some of the culinary delights that Pollenca and Alcudia have to offer. I would be testing Monday and Thursday, doing a regular pig visit on the Tuesday. I walked on the farm; one I had never been too to be greeted by "You must be Martin's brother?" A farm where my twin had visited many times in his capacity in selling farm machinery.

Mallorca was very enjoyable, a great break and lovely to be back helping Mick revive the old drive to their house we had discovered two years previously, pre-Covid, under brambles, overgrown olives, bamboo, and other thorny trees. The mosquitoes had not gone away either and found me just as tasty as the years previously. They, Mick and Jill, had rented out some of their land to a local shepherd, my veterinary eye was needed to be cast over his nineteen sheep, some of which were lame. This soon became eighteen!

I had two more weeks of Tb testing to do before I finished my stint, my first day back being a really busy one. Two sizable beef herds then finishing with a small test of some British Whites, who like the Longhorns, know what to do with their horns.

An early start testing pedigree Limousins which included blood testing them as well for the herd to maintain its high health status. The farmers here were good friends and had requested me to do the test as I was happy to do both Tb and blood test myself. It was quite sad for me that having done their test for so many years that this really would be the last time I would be doing it for them.

One last week to go, two incredibly early starts then back to retirement. Both these tests were on farms I had enjoyed working on, only for me to be informed that on the Monday test, firstly that Animal Health would be blood testing the cattle at the same time, a Gamma Interferon test looking for Tb that doesn't always show up on the skin test, and secondly the farmer had Covid but was going to stay out of the way.

I arrived on the farm to be greeted by the farmer! Though he did try and keep his distance, and one of the testers informed me that she also had just recovered from the disease. It was a slow test, I had to help with some of the bleeding when they could not find a vein. We had nearly finished when someone came around the corner where we were testing to ask if anyone had a greyish car. I did, one of the testers did. A delivery lorry had just arrived and in reversing, had hit one of the cars.

It was mine! When I had finished the test, I inspected the damage. A whole line of cars and he had hit mine. Was I jinked with these cars? You did not need to be a garage engineer to know this was a new bonnet and headlight unit. Thankfully, liability was admitted, and the car was repaired at a later date.

My last test, and sadly because again the farmers were good friends, I had my only reactor in all that time I had been testing. Two beautiful, well grown heifers that were due to calve in three months' time. If that test had been clear, this farm would have gone out of short interval testing, now they were back to square one and they too would be having a Gamma Interferon test done. Thankfully at the time of writing they are now clear and have been now for over six months.

Back to retirement again though I had said I would do one week in mid-December doing one large farm, a test of nearly eight hundred cattle split over two days.

But my father whose dementia was deteriorating by the day, took a turn for the worse and I spent nearly a week looking after him along with a close friend, sure that he would not see the next day, then the next. Having to watch over him all night as he became bed-ridden other than occasional periods of aggression, obstinance. It was heart breaking see such a great man like this. And then on the fifth day of this, while talking to the visiting nurse, he did manage to summon enough strength to get up but then fall over and crack his head open on the tiled floor. We know enough of ambulance waiting times at hospitals, I spent a long night at A &E hoping someone could help me deal with him while awaiting results of scans, physically having to restrain him as he wanted to get up again but should not with a head injury.

He never came home again, eventually being transferred into a care home before dying in hospital with respiratory complications.

It did mean though that by the time I had completed the following weeks testing, I had done enough. I was exhausted looking after dad, worrying and emotionally strained. These early starts were not helping. That was going to be the last Tb test I would do as I have mentioned earlier, and I think I was quite relieved.

If nothing else over those past few weeks I had met some very pleasant farmers, had revisited past acquaintances and had been given the chance to see some of my ex-work colleagues, especially Cristina and Alex, and of course Siobhan and Charlotte. It was always a pleasure to see those two. But even in those few months since I had left, what a change in personnel there had been, I hardly recognised anybody in the office now.

In the beginning of December 2021, Avian Influenza had reared its ugly head in our area and I had previously been asked by my former employers if I would be prepared to do work for them if Animal Health called upon them for their services, something they had an obligation to do. In January 2022 I was working again, starting from a base just outside Leominster dealing with outbreaks in Newent, Gloucestershire and in the Leominster area. I would receive a briefing of my duties at the same time as a health and Safety seminar, necessary to perform my duties. What organisation, I did one on my phone while watching the other on a laptop in the village hall, our base. Then it was off to do my first calls inspecting backyard poultry flocks to check there were no signs of disease in Protection Zones close to where there had been infected premises.

I had a two-hour journey down to Newent where I would be expected on my first day to visit seven different premises, luckily all very close to each other. We were kitted out as in my previous experience of Avian Flu in 2017 with protective clothing, gloves, respirators, and plenty of Virkon, the disinfectant we would be using in the outbreak. We were to check for signs of disease, on biosecurity and the potential risks of each premises for possible infection, giving appropriate advice where necessary.

One did feel that one was taking more precautions than a nurse working in an intensive care ward in a Covid unit, but that was what APHA decreed so that is what was done.

Most people were extremely pleased to see us, accept our advice but wondering when restrictions for the disease would be lifted. Sadly, that was something we could not advise on, that decision was for APHA when they felt it fit to do so.

The demanding work though was not the visits but all the paperwork one had to do afterwards and then submit to control. My first day, I think I finished my last report just before midnight. At eight thirty the next morning I would be back at base getting my instructions for that day, taking me back down to Newent for another seven visits, another tiring day and late night doing the reporting. But for the first week in January the weather was surprisingly mild, a day of sunshine and it was a pleasure to be outside and to be meeting a variety of different and interesting people, but again concerned with when their chickens could go outside and when they could sell their eggs again. These birds were used to an outdoor life and were getting stressed with their confinement which if like 2021, could last until April at least.

The following day was quieter but showed some of the inefficiency of the whole project. We had five vets waiting for briefings at the village hall which was our HQ but no sign of anybody from APHA. Two of those vets were new on the case and needed a full briefing as to their duties plus their health and Safety, and to be supplied with equipment. Nobody arrived. I was supposed to be handing over all the reports I had written to somebody, but again nobody was there.

I had one surveillance visit to do up the road, about ten

minutes away but when completed, now midday, still no-one had arrived to give these two vets their initiation, and one was supposed to be in Newent after lunch.

I briefed them as best as I could about filling in the paperwork and supplying them with what kit I could spare. At last, someone did arrive, I was able to hand over my reports and the other two were at last sent on their way.

We found out that allocations had now transferred from APHA to XLVets Farmcare, hopefully this would make the ship run more efficiently though we still had to pre- and post-brief to APHA vets, most of whom were foreign, and it did take a bit of time to bridge the language barriers. But over the course of my time doing bird flu, I found several of them lovely and would always try to make them my point of contact.

My fourth day was an interesting day, again down near Newent, but not because of Avian Influenza but because of the places and people I met. My first call saw me arriving at a rather spectacular mansion, very Elizabethan in style and there were obviously a lot of renovations going on. I did the bird business and then over a cup of coffee with the lady of the house, a delightful young woman, we were able to have a chat about the property. It showed I was in the wrong profession, this house, a Harley Street dermatologist owned these grounds. He employed two full time builders on the property while slowly renovating it to how he and his wife wanted. Such considerations as taking down old internal walls to find bats there and work would stop until the bats had relocated. So much history in one building that I am sure a book could have been written on it.

I had finished my assigned calls and checking in to base was asked if I could do one more call, but it would mean a cold call if I could not contact them by phone. I tried but was unable to so arrived at this premises and knocked on the front door. It was answered by a man who looked all too familiar to me. How many people do you recognise from their ears, and it was not Mr Spock who had just answered the door.

What a stupid question I asked him, though I guess if I had been given the right spelling of his name, I would have known the answer already.

"You're a rugby player?" I asked.

"Yes."

Standing in front of me was a former England and British Lion rugby player, indeed a captain of them. I apologised for the cold call but explained what we were having to do in the area as it was near to an infected premises. I inspected his flock of birds and would have to account for the one that the dog had got and then we got on to talking about rugby, some vets he had known and about depression. I was a little in awe of him as an international, had read his autobiography in the past but he was such an easy person to talk to as he told me of some of his lows, and was fascinated about my history, of climbing Kilimanjaro to get over my depression. It was a turnaround in that he was interested in my personal battles and overcoming them. He asked me in for a coffee, I wish I had accepted as I would have loved the conversation to continue, but I was all too aware of the time pressures of getting home and writing these damn reports. It was a pleasure to meet him and the news that I had met someone famous soon spread around APHA after my debriefing.

I had another week of these short visits, taking me to Newent, Wem and Hay on Wye, a town I had always wanted to visit, but on a dreary day I did not stop long. I had finished a two-week stint and would have to say that it paid very well, now I had a couple of private visits to do, a pig inspection again and a blood test, and my time was my own.

Jane and I at last took the break we had planned back in December before my father was taken ill, a long weekend in Llandudno again to see what the place was like in winter. But at the end of the trip was when dad was admitted to hospital, and he died a week later.

I needed a distraction; it would be another five weeks before we could arrange the funeral for all the family to be there, so was quite grateful to be contacted again to do Surveillance visits on some large poultry units near Ross on Wye. This I found really interesting, seeing a side of the industry I had had little to do with throughout my career. We were not talking of one, five, ten birds on a premises but now a quarter or half a million birds. The technology, environmental control, the biosecurity, just how the complete process worked was new to me and I found fascinating. I suppose this could be deemed as factory farming, but I found the care and welfare given by the workers on these units to be more than satisfactory. I found them all to be very conscientious in what they did and ended up having no worries about this type of farming.

These duties I continued with through March and early April, visiting some exceptionally large units and then a couple of turkey producers. I also saw the egg production side of the industry and hatcheries. I even visited, small world, someone whose cattle farm I had visited all those years ago when I worked in the Forest of Dean and had travelled to Canada with one of my old mates. Another farmer, one of the turkey farmers, also had a large dairy herd and I spent a fascinating hour talking cows with him once I had finished the task for what I was actually there for.

We had hoped we had got on top of the outbreak in our region, and it had certainly given me some work and income.

In May I would be called upon to go and check some young quails in a house in Wolverhampton, a tracing visit to check for possible infection in birds from hatched eggs. A delicate task to take oral swabs from these young birds no bigger than a hen's egg and perhaps it did seem like overkill to dress up in all the kit we were expected to do to go into this young lady's kitchen, but that is what we had to do.

Another call near Malvern to check on two hens, and I personally would find it hard to justify the expense of this visit, but rules are rules, so it had to be done. I would question going forward whether the expense for this Notifiable disease can continue, infection is so inherent in the wild bird population that it may now be the case that we just have to live with it. I have seen in turkey flocks how it can decimate numbers so quickly, but in these large units, their biosecurity should be good enough against the introduction of all bird disease.

I had decided that was enough. As the first anniversary of retirement fast approached, I had worked a lot, and had enjoyed it but without the commitment of having to turn out every day. To be "bird clean", I would only do a visit every third or fourth day so could very much arrange them to suit me. Now was the time to explore other of my interests, starting with a long-awaited trip to Malta, the one I had planned for straight after retirement but never did because of the complications of Covid.

It was a great trip, seeing much of the island and would have been made perfect if we could have seen *Carmen* in open air theatre in Valetta, but we were a week too early.

A year had passed since retirement, a busy year and now time to move on.

A LONG GOODNIGHT:

I S THIS THE place to end my story, time to say goodnight after a long, much longer than intended career as a farm vet. Well, perhaps not yet but we are approaching the end. So having started this tale early one Sunday morning, then perhaps the place to finish it is as we draw into the evening hours, going into and through the night.

Here, I would have to say though the modern vet seems reluctant to do night and weekend calls, and I can appreciate the impact it has on a work/life balance, then I have throughout my career actually enjoyed a lot of it. Yes, I can agree that there have been many times when that work in what we shall call antisocial hours has been a pain in the backside, an inconvenience. This has been especially so when trying to decide with friends to do something, visit those who are some distance away, go on theatre trips, the list is endless. But I have always accepted it as part of the job, or should I say vocation again, although it was nice when it did not happen too often. Having said that, did I have a sense of guilt in my last few months when I stopped doing nights and weekends? No, I was quite relieved, and any guilt was reduced by the fact I was not being paid so much because I had made the decision to stop this work. Age was catching up on me.

But did I miss it, or do I miss it now? A definite no to that question with a big BUT that I do miss some of the type of work that I did out of hours. The lambings, the calvings, even those tiring calls when you were trying to put a cow's "bed" back in, and the camaraderie one developed with the farmers while doing his work. Yes, I do miss some of that and although I have done calvings since retirement, I definitely have missed the lambings in springtime, that part of the year that one sees the start of new life, rebirth of the countryside. It was always very satisfying to bring a new lamb, even better twins, into this world even in the middle of the night. Whether visiting a lambing shed on a farm or meeting the farmer with his truck containing a pregnant ewe at the surgery under a moonlit sky, seeing farmer, ewe and lamb all depart happy was a very satisfying feeling, and that would have occurred many times throughout my career as a farm vet.

Large animal work tends to be a bit seasonal, especially out of hours work. Summer has always tended to be abit quieter, usually most of the stock is outside on grass so stocking densities are less than when housed so individual stress should be less. Spring is the time of lambing for most people though over the past few years we do seem to be carrying them out increasingly anytime from mid-December until late May. Calving in my early days was an all the year round issue but now the majority of dairy farms are either autumn or spring block calvers, making management of these high performance milk producers easier, and even beef cattle now tend to have their calving pattern concentrated so that all the calves can be weaned together when they should be of equal size. Again, there is a management advantage to this. Winter for pneumonia problems, summer for parasite problems, but herd problems like this will generally be dealt with during the day.

If one actually breaks down our working day, office hours of say eight, eight fifteen until five, five thirty, then it means that nearly sixty per cent of the day is covered by the out of hours rota, working alone or with the help of a backup if needed. This is a long time to cover, and I cannot think of many of all those nights I have done when I have not been called out. Early evening when milking is going on or coming to an end, and likewise d from five in the morning when the next milking is taking place, all cows will be observed at this time and there is the potential that the on-duty vet may get called out to see a sick cow.

But I guess, especially in winter when the hours of daylight are much reduced, then once one gets home it is nice to think the evening is your own and you will not get disturbed. Even more so when it is chucking it down with rain, a snowstorm is whipped up, a blizzard to drive through, there is a howling gale, or the temperature is starting to plummet well below zero. A lovely thought that you can shut the door behind you and keep in the warm! Conversely, in summer it is nice sometimes to get out especially if there is a spectacular sunset to see while you are driving to a call. The freshness, the greens of late spring, the blossom on the trees and the acres and acres of yellow stretching before you as the oilseed rape comes into flower.

So, the phones would be put through to ever took the evening calls when the office shut, earlier in my career to a partner in the practice, my wife, an outside agency, but more lately to me, to my own work mobile. I would have to answer the calls and do them, only hoping that no-one would ring while I was engaged up a cow's backside or in the middle of a caesarean. And, if there were any calls it would be for a sick cow or calf seen at milking time, or from one of those dear small holders who had just got home from work and gone out to look at their stock. Some of those calls would just be giving advice, some would be attending a case which was not really an emergency but then they would be at work the following day as well. You just had to accept that some of these calls would have to be seen out of hours, which is the service we offered! And there would be a number of calls that could have been seen earlier in the day, or yesterday, or the day before that but had just been left and left. They were always the frustrating calls, being called out when the prognosis was getting poorer and poorer, the outcome was disappointing and how many of these callouts were by farmers who were bad at paying their bills!

One of the more exciting callouts at or after milking time was for a cow that had cut her teat, or more excitingly sometimes, cut her milk vein, that large blood vessel running forward from the udder towards the front of the cow. What one could say was that if the vein was cut or nicked, then it bled profusely with a jet of blood spraying out over some distance. You would arrive on the farm to find the farmer or a helper valiantly holding a pressure pad over the bleeder until we, the professional help arrived.

Of course the exciting part of this and of cut teats was that you were having to work at the kicking end of the cow, she not taking kindly to a stranger coming up and poking around an area that has been previously injured by a nasty cut or another cow standing on the teat and tearing it in a bad way. The old Abreast parlours were great because the cow was standing on a raised platform where she was milked, me the vet below her and so close to that lethal weapon, her back feet. We could try lifting that leg and tying it out of the way but invariably there would still be enough movement in the leg that me the poor vet was still vulnerable.

Of course we would give a local anaesthetic to the affected area before doing anything to it, a nice ring block around the top of the teat to numb it, but this meant sticking a needle in several times, however fine it may be, and if the teat is swollen which it often is if it has been trodden on, then it makes it harder to get local in through an fine needle. Herring Bone parlours were even more fun because here you would often be working behind the cow so there were two weapons that she could aim at you. There were cunning kick bars which fit over the back of the cow, down to in front of the udder so that if she bends her back to kick it gives her a lot of discomfort, holding the cow's tail up vertically will, have a similar affect t but means someone has to perch themselves behind the cow somehow to do it.

Once the local was administered, things did get a lot easier and we, the vets would carefully try to sew the skin edges back together, making sure the milk canal was intact as well. We did not want milk leaking through the wound when it was sutured closed. In olden days we would have big needles with nylon which we had to thread through and when the wound was closed, one had all these big horrid knots but thanks to the medical profession, some of the kinder suture materials were developed and came into veterinary use, and even better, already had a needle on them, a fine needle at that. Materials such as silk I started to use, so soft but if it had one fault it was if it was the same colour as the cow. Trying to tie off sutures when the material is so fine, is not easy when it blends into the background colour scheme and the patient has taken a dislike to you as well. And in ageing years, the eyesight is not what it was previously. But we persevered and invariably managed to salvage the teat so the cow could carry on producing milk through it as long as it was a cut that could be sutured, vertical cuts great, but horizontal cuts and the blood supply to the lower edge would be compromised and they wound would break down. With these ones then often, it would be a matter of trimming the teat to the best anatomical shape you could produce that would allow the cow to be milked easily.

But if these fine suture materials were welcome, even better followed when we started to staple wounds, easily bringing the edges of wounds together, producing a nice, neat closure and then there was a little instrument that would make their removal easy at the appropriate time. These staples were also wonderful for suturing the small wounds over milk veins that I had previously mentioned, saving having to open over the blood vessel to try to find the bleeding point and closing it. Stapling over it seemed to produce enough pressure that the wound would stop haemorrhaging. And even better still, I had in my small animal days, or at the end of them, started gluing small wounds. Cleaning up the wound and trying to stop any bleeders, then applying glue down either side of the wound and bringing the edges together, especially in operations like routine bitch spays, produced a wonderfully neat wound closure.

I started to use it in these cut teats, and it worked well as long as I had some on me, as long as the cow restraint was good enough that you could hold the edges together without having to keep letting go because of swinging feet. And of course, if I, the vet, did not get stuck to the cow's teat myself. The wounds healed beautifully, were easy to milk, and there were no stitches or staples to remove. The only frustration would be that, not using this technique that often, one hoped that when you got your superglue out to use, one hoped it had not already set in its tube.

Once early evening was out of the way, then we basically turn into obstetricians. Calvings, lambings, farrowing's, become our trade.

How many times in those long nights have I been called out to farrow a pig. Not many through my career but then where I have worked have not been big pig keeping areas. So, despite being classed as the pig vet in the practice, delivering piglets has been few and far between. But then, unless you have along thin arm, there is not a long you can do. The advantage of a farrowing crate is that the sow is well restrained, and it is usually obvious when her time has come to produce, as we were taught at university, three months, three weeks, and three days after being served. There is a drug you can give to induce farrowing so that if you have a batch of sows due, you can manipulate the event more into social hours, but the units I have dealt with did not have the numbers to justify that.

A keen eye by the pigman and if no progress, or the sow produces one or two piglets then stops, then I would be called out to assist. I have got a thin and long arm, but the anatomy of the pig's uterus is such that you cannot just reach in and feel all the piglets with your hand. The uterus has two long and convoluted horns to it, so it is quite possible that you can feel piglets, but you are only feeling them through the wall of the uterus. They are some distance from being assessable to me. If you bear in mind that a sow could produce up to twenty plus piglets at one go, then there is quite a traffic jam of piglets waiting to come out. All I can do unless I am able to reach a piglet or two with my fingers and pull them out is to give a shot of Oxytocin which will make the uterus contract and move the piglets along. It is very quick acting, and you can see the results, the sow starting to strain again within minutes. Time to have another feel inside and hopefully remove another piglet. If the process is working, then they should be moving further towards the outside world and will either be delivered my mum pushing, or with a further human helping hand.

Oxytocin injections can be repeated if necessary, and although the majority of farrowings I have been to the litter has been small (which may mean a big piglet has blocked the passage), the injections have always worked. I have never had to Caesar a pig, sedation, anaesthesia can be an issue.

Piglets are cute little things when born and will soon be up and walking about trying to find a teat to suckle. Bu often if there has been a problem, the piglets that the vet delivers are dead, they have been stuck and died in the process of birth.

For us the vets, there is always one plus and one minus. Piglets require heat so you will never be cold doing a farrowing, even in winter as there will be an infra-red light handy to warm them and maintain their body temperatures. The downside, when you get home, however much you try, you smell of pig and it is not the easiest smell to get rid of.

Spring is the time of lambing, and it is still a joy to me to be driving round over those months of march, April, and May to see young lambs frolicking around the fields in the throes of warming sunshine as we move towards our warmer months. Running around in bunches, hopping, skipping, and jumping upon mum's back as she is lying down, "I'm king of the castle" with the lamb's twin.

Lambing time, one had always to accept the good with the bad, not every delivery would produce one, two, three live lambs. There would be those ewes that aborted, lambed early and these invariably had dead lambs or if they were alive, they had no vitality, their bodies were not sufficiently developed to cope with life ex-utero. Those ewes that had suffered from twin lamb disease and the body had made the decision, sacrifice the lambs or oneself. A couple of the vets decided year in, year out that they would hold a sweep to see who lambed the most live lambs, I never entered my figures. It was the luck of the draw what lambing you attended and if you went to one that produced dead triplets and they had been dead for a while, that greatly impacted on your "score".

But in the late evening, middle of the night, it was never an issue for me to get up and go out to do a lambing unless I was forewarned that it was going to be for dead and smelly lambs. Evening heading off in the snow sometimes under a dark night sky, peering through the windscreen to pick out the road, it was a pleasure to arrive at a farm, enter the barn and find the ewe that needed attention in her pen. A bucket of warm (sometimes too hot) water was provided, and kneeling down behind the ewe one would insert a hand to find what the trouble with the lambing was, an over large lamb, tangled up twins or sometimes, it was just a straightforward delivery. Things can alter a lot in the time taken from the call out to arrival on the farm. But as with calvings, it is always better to get called out too early than too late!

I was ready to start my obstetrical examination and with that hand inserted inside to reproductive tract of the ewe, what would I find? Most sheep farmers have their ewes scanned so they know almost a hundred percent how many lambs will be inside the ewe. Scanning is a great aid to management of the pregnant ewe, so that her nutrition can be managed properly especially if she is carrying twins or triplets which have a huge demand on her energy resources, especially in winter when pregnancy occurs when the value of grass at pasture is limited. So, at that initial examination I will be given an idea how many lambs will be inside, and the more experienced shepherds will tell me what they think the problem is with the lambing.

But that information may not be correct always. It would be many times that I have been told there are twins, and they are coming backwards only to find when I put my hand inside, I feel one, two heads! Or vice versa, its coming normally but the lamb's head is turned back only to find that I am feeling hind legs. So that initial examination is always important for me to ascertain what the problem is, how many legs are being presented at the same time, two, three, even four or five. How many heads, if any at all, and sometimes it may just be a tail that is presented. More unusually, it may be intestines that are showing, are they the lambs or has mum ruptured her uterus and it is her own guts coming out, a hopeless scenario.

I have assessed the problem and am ready to start trying to lamb the ewe. Here patience is a virtue while trying to work out which legs belong to which lambs and then in untangling them, removing the lamb by gentle traction through the birth canal. Then, hopefully, that satisfying moment when having brought the lamb out into the outside world, giving its chest a rub, the shake of the lamb's head, a splutter as it tries to clear its airway and then takes its first breath. Success! Then re-entering the birth canal to remove a twin, and again if there is a triplet to deliver. Complications like the head being back, turned the wrong way inside the ewe's uterus can sometimes be hard to correct, especially if the uterus is starting to contract down, finding hind legs if only the tail is presented likewise. This is a true breach, and one often must push the lamb back into the uterus to have enough room to correct the presentation and have the back legs in the correct position to deliver the lamb.

But again, always checking after the last lamb has been delivered that there is not another still inside, then I can admire my work with hopefully the live lambs which mum is now desperate to deal with. It is very satisfying, especially deep into the night.

Some of these lambings may be because the farmer's hands are just too big for lambing, some because they are inexperienced, and we often held lambing courses to try and educate especially small holders and young farmers into the art of lambing. Others would even take time for us as experienced lambers and vets to sort out, and of course some we would make the decision that the only way the lambs were going to come out would be if they were removed through the side, a caesarean.

I have described one earlier, and again it is a satisfying op to be able to remove two live lambs and when finished suturing the hole up, being able to present mum with her new family. And with her strong maternal instincts she is only too keen to start mothering, licking them clean. A beautiful thing of nature, that instinct.

Paul, who I have mentioned earlier, flushed a lot of his ewes, implanting embryos into them so produce high genetic merit pedigree lambs. These were valuable, would generally lamb in a very short interval and so for a few days when they were due to lamb we would be on stand-by to be there and often to perform a caesarean. It was only down the road for me, I could get the call, get dressed at night and be there in less than twenty minutes. Paul had a really good sheep shed with a room attached where he had bought his own operating table, it was well kitted out for us to perform this operation in the best of conditions. At one time he had a shepherd called Aled working for him and when called out he would greet me with the ewe ready for me to examine and start operating if necessary (if he said caesarean then it almost always was) We would secure the ewe on the table, get her clipped up and I would get underway with the operation. He had rigged up a tv over the operating table so while he helped quieten the ewe, he would catch up on all the shows he wanted to watch while I beavered away at delivering a lamb.

The system worked well, and often it would not be much over an hour, having carried out an operation and cleaned up again, that I could be getting back into bed again, hoping I wouldn't get disturbed again. But at its busiest, I could often be back helping Aled or Paul with another lambing, another caesarean not too long afterwards again.

But the key was that we intervened early so could always make the correct decision, leave it little longer or operate so a successful outcome could be achieved.

Yes, I do miss lambing time.

Calvings are similar but obviously on a larger scale, and there are not as many cattle in the country as there are sheep. With students with me, I often wondered how you can teach them properly to calve a cow as the farmer does not want a student interfering, risking the loss of a potential calf. I guess lambings give them a good start as to the potential problems, the rest comes down to a bigger size, strength and needing longer arms.

But the same problems arise in birth and the routine would be the same, even late at night, early morning. I knew if I got called out of bed then it would be longer before I was back tucked up again, but as long as I knew there was every chance that a live calf could be produced, then I did not mind going out. The procedure would be the same, the farmer or cowman would tell me what he had found and was usually right although on more than one occasion, even with a calf, the calf coming backwards was actually coming forwards and vice versa. One leg, two or three legs, no legs but a head, and again guts which would indicate the likelihood of the calf being a schistosome, it was grossly deformed.

One was lucky if one got a bucket of water, unlike when I first started as a vet, unless you asked and then it was often cold which was great in the middle of a freezing night. My examination would reveal what the problem in calving really was and then it was time to get down to it and try and get the calf out. Some of these calves would be massive and would take time, patience, and a lot of lubrication to bring it out into the world, taking care not to damage mum in the process. Obviously, labour can be in short supply in the middle of the night and here the calving aid, used properly, was a great benefit probably doing the work of two or three men. The presentation of the calf would need to be corrected, retrieving a leg or the head, which was pointing in the wrong direction, or in a true breech, both back legs. Here you would have to push the calf back in, and hard to describe how one did it, push part of it back while trying to grab its lower limbs and pull them back towards you. A lot of sweat in my years as a vet would have been passed doing his, calving cows.

But eventually, success and the calf would be delivered from the cow and into this world, sometimes coming with a rush at the end, so that we fell backwards pulling and when it did come, it landed on top of us as we fell.

Obviously, some of those calvings turned out to be caesareans as in sheep, and the operation took a lot longer than in a sheep. Rigging up adequate lighting was always a trial, and especially in my early days, how many of these c-sections would I have done in semi-darkness in old cowsheds with inadequate light. That is when I had to get used to cut fingers after an op because I could not see well enough where my hands were when operating, especially if inside the cow. Sometimes it was me that I cut!

But I had some really interesting conversations about anything and everything in those midnight hours while delivering a calf one way or another. It was very satisfying, even if in the night the journeys could be long and in winter, hazardous. Those early days in Devon when I would travel fifteen miles maximum, and before I retired when that journey could be forty, fifty miles each way.

Washing in the dark was not easy either, often getting home thinking you were clean only to find that you still had blood and foetal fluids over your arms and your face. On more than one occasion when back home, looking in a mirror I thought myself lucky I had not been stopped by the police on the way home, I would have looked like an axe murderer. And when I got up in the morning and went out to the car to find where I had leant over, delving into the boot or the backseat, there was blood all over the paintwork of the car as well.

But again, it is, was, so satisfying delivering a new life into this world, whatever hour of the day it was. I think my best (or worst whichever way one wants to look at it) night I went out five times, but five live calves made it all worthwhile.

The other joy was the journey. If going I would be thinking of the task at hand, then returning home, if I was not battling a blizzard or fog, then I could enjoy the nature of the night. The sunsets over the Welsh hills as I travelled west, the sunrises in Devon over Hembury Fort, or in Shropshire those magnificent skies witnessed as the sun rose behind the Wrekin. The reflections of sunrays on the Severn as I crossed it near Atcham, the mists rising from the river on early summer mornings. The emergence of spring, of May blossom at the sides of the roads at dawn. Barn owls on their nightly food collections, foxes trotting along the sides of the roads, and the occasional badger cubs playing near roadside. I have loved nature, and this is the time to see it, when wildlife has the countryside to themselves. A real joy to me.

So much to see and do and to appreciate of our rural landscape. So much on those long, good nights that has made my job so fulfilling, and something that I will miss.

BACK in an OLD ROUTINE:

O VER THE PAST few months, late winter, and the spring of 2022 I had regularly helped out on Bob's farm at Windy Meadows. Whether it had been helping at his Tb tests, blood sampling for his High Health status or to see the odd sick animal or two, when needed then Bob had been on the phone to me asking me for assistance.

If I thought I had calved my last cow when I walked out of the office into retirement in 2021, then I was mistaken. 2022, another calving season about to begin and it was not long before I got my first call for assistance, though what Bob called me for was not a calving but to remove the afterbirth from a cow that had calved a week earlier. This would be a smelly job, even more so when examining the cow per vagina, the first thing I felt was another calf. And the odour emanating from the rear end of the cow was foul. I did manage to get the calf out, dead and rotting by this time but had to warn that the cow was toxic, and chances of recovery were not great.

Thankfully, the next cow calved normally by herself though after a few days it did seem when I was asked to look at it as if the calf had some sort of joint disease. We had seen a couple of calves like this the previous year. I went to calve another cow then another, and it was evident that something was amiss as one of these and another couple that had calved normally were too showing signs of joint deformity. It was to the internet that I looked for an answer, suspecting a degree of copper deficiency, but looking closer thinking it more a Manganese deficiency. A combination of bought in red clover silage and his water supply was probably contributing to this problem but at least now we could do something about it with supplementing the mineral into the water for the cows and injecting all calves at birth to boost their mineral levels. Thankfully all but the first calf were soon walking normally with no sign of the joint disease that they had been born with.

But my calving skills were required on more than one occasion as the spring progressed, even on one evening when asked to assist, I arrived on the farm to have to calve a black cow in the dark with only my head torch to assist me. Successfully completed and having dropped the calf gently from mum into our maternity ambulance, a wheelbarrow to take it to a box with a nice deep bed, and reunite it with mum, Bob did one last check around the cow shed to make sure all the other cows were okay. Another was calving, and again with much difficulty in the dark with no light and chasing this black cow, we did manage to get her out of the yard and into the cattle crush to examine her. She was ready to calve and after a bit of manipulation I was able to drop the next calf gently into the barrow which Bob had now retrieved again. Off he trundled with the calf, injecting this one and the one I had just delivered with their mineral jab.

I do not know why but intuition told me there was another calf still inside this cow, one should always check anyway. But here, I expected to find a twin, a gut feeling. Yes, there was a second which felt a bigger calf than number one and was a bit more of a struggle to bring into the world. I had called to Bob to bring back the wheelbarrow and we were soon wheeling this second calf to join its twin, then we let mum join them. A surprise for her in the dark to find not one but two healthy young calves to rear. Interestingly at a later date we found one to be suffering mildly with the joint problem we had seen in earlier calves, but on a second injection it made an uneventful recovery.

After three live calves in an evening, a glass of red was a suitable reward before returning home and after a good wash, a not very warm me snuggling back into bed next to my sleeping wife!

Bob had decided over the course of time that it was time to give up on his farming. He wasn't getting any younger, had staff problems, his latest helper who was a bit of a know-it-all had just demolished one of his sheds with a fore loader, and was worried what would happen if something happened to him, his lovely wife Venessa certainly could not manage the farm and the animals.

We knew this was going to be his last calving season, then in the early autumn he would have a dispersal sale of his pedigree herd up in Carlisle. I was a pleasure to help him out where I could, partly out of interest and partly as he had always been good to me, it was a chance to pay back something to him. How many calvings did I end up doing in this calving season, probably a dozen. But the odd stillborn calf, and one or two which we struggled to get going either because they would not suckle by themselves or because mum did not have a lot of milk; you could see it was starting to get him down. One cow, possessive of her calf, went for him, pinning him down. Another calf we struggled with died in my arms as we tried to get fluids into it. Bob was visibly upset, tears in his eyes.

I had arranged to go to Malta for a week but told Bob he too needed to get away, he should take himself and Venessa off to his beloved Italy. Their plans over the previous two years had been upset by Covid, they were fully vaccinated, Italy was open. THEY SHOULD GO!

He gave in and finally decided to go to Italy as it happened the day after we returned from Malta. I had previously said any help he needed while he was away, do not hesitate to ask me. I could keep an eye on the place. He arranged for a friend of his to house sit while they were away, Pete his new workman could call me if necessary.

A week or so before they went to Malta we went for barbeque at Bob's, along with his son and grandchild, and a couple of friends, the ones in fact who were going to look after the house. Over a glass of wine or two, the husband asked me firstly if Bob always followed my advice. I tried to explain that whatever I suggested, if it worked then everyone would be happy. If it went wrong, then it would be

Bob who would have to foot the bill and the consequences. He had stuck with me for over thirty years so I hoped he had trust in me, so "yes, he would usually do what I suggested". His next question was to ask me if I thought it was right for Bob to sell up now.

A slightly harder question in that knowing what Bob had gone through in the past, knowing his attention to detail in his breeding policies for his pedigree herd and knowing how it was now affecting him and with him looking to the future, especially if something unforeseen were to happen to him, then my answer was yes. But I said that there had to be a proviso to this question. So many farmers only interest is their farm which is all time consuming. If they meet anyone else, they talk farming. They live and breathe farming. If that farm suddenly goes, what are they going to do with their time, they may not have any other hobbies.

So, my answer was yes provided that Bob found other interests, it was time for new beginnings for him, and for Venessa.

Bob was beginning to have second thoughts about leaving the farm and leaving it in the hands of this other couple who had no farming background and were frail themselves. They too were slightly concerned about leaving their family home and their cat. As we were departing from the barbeque, Jane and I said to both Bob and Venessa, if they had any worries then we would be quite happy to come over and look after the place ourselves for the twelve days, a change of scenery would be nice.

Our passing words were "Think about it, we were quite happy to help if they wanted us to."

I got a phone call from Bob the next morning, he and Venessa had thought about it and would be happier if Jane and I would be looking after the farm while they were away. If we had time that day, could we pop over and they would show what was what in terms of feeding the cattle, what was due to calve, there was one animal that needed to leave the farm while they were away. Venessa would show Jane where everything was in the house that we might need. They were far happier with that arrangement, and I would be able to guide his normal worker who just came in for a couple of hours in the morning, and I would be there to do the afternoon feeding.

I was going to be a farmer again, back to my roots! I was excited.

Our cross over was that we arrived back from Malta on the Monday evening, Bob and Venessa were heading the opposite way later that night to park their car up at Manchester Airport and fly to Italy. We had gone Ryanair, I admit not by choice but at a time of airport hold-ups at least they were flying, and on time. Bob and Venessa, easyJet, and they did get held up, but at least they were gone and would get a much-needed break.

I did not need to be at the farm until the following afternoon as Pete would have dealt with the cattle that morning. We arrived in two cars; I would still need to travel back to Telford every other day to deal with my garden and especially my tomato plants. Venessa had left a list of instructions and there was a fridge full of food that needed consuming before its expiry date, including a few rather nice-looking steaks. We would be lighting the barbeque in due course to enjoy these.

I knew what I was supposed to be doing and which cows I should be looking out for calving. That afternoon I would start my feeding duties and do my evening check around all the cattle. I took in all the thistles that were standing in each field, they were going to go, or as many as I could get round with a scythe.

Having done my rounds, I cooked tea for us, and we settled down in our "new home" for the evening. A lovely house overlooking some of Bob's land and certainly from upstairs one had a panoramic view of the whole farm and all the cattle, a view that extended to beyond Telford and the Wrekin.

I knew that one cow was due to calve imminently, what her ear number was to identify her but had also been warned that this cow more than any other in the herd was a very possessive mother and that when she calved, watch out for her. If you tried to do anything to the calf, well she would not let you, she would go for you. Lucky us looking after her!

This was a week where extreme heat was forecast,

temperatures that could break records. Little rain had fallen recently, and grass growth was poor to no growth at all, and certainly on the non-peat land, the fields were slowly burning up, the grass turning yellow what little there was. If there was any grass in these fields, it tended to be hidden by the thistles.

What it did mean though was that we had some glorious sunsets during our stay. Having watched the sun go down we retired to bed, the first night of our farming sojourn.

I was up early and could survey the cows next to the house through the bedroom window. They were mostly gathered around the gateway either expecting to move to a slightly better pasture or awaiting to have their hay racks topped up. With the dispersal sale less than twelve weeks away we were having to supplement their feed as grass was short and they needed to be in good condition, sale condition. All seemed content and no sign of any water bags to suggest any cow may be going into labour.

I went outside to do my feeding, a couple of groups of heifers and bulls, Pete would feed the cows when he arrived because he could use the tractor and fore loader. It was many years since I had to drive one and they had changed a lot over that time.

I had my breakfast then went on my morning check of all the cattle. As I passed the cows, I thought that I could now see a water bag visible from the rear end of one cow. I had not seen anything earlier so the cow could only be in early first stage labour, I would give her more time and by then if I needed to calve her, or at least examine her, Pete would have arrived plus another who helped, another Bob.

I went back an hour later and there seemed little progress. We would have to get her in which involved separating her from the other cows all of whom really wanted now top leave this field for pastures new, more grazing. We did manage to get her out with only a couple of others, then return them back to the field. We had her in the yard, but would she co-operate and go into the race and then the crush, she wanted to be back with her mates. Her temperament was turning out to be just what Bob had warned me of. In the end we had to mix her with a group of young bulls that were in a yard and get them all to go through the race. She was happy to follow them, we had her at last so I could examine her.

I put my overalls on, it was hot enough without them, and examined her per vagina. She was ready to calve, but I could feel two big feet and a large head waiting to come out. The calf was slightly twisted as well. Helper Bob was there to help we while Pete continued with the feeding. This was going to be a struggle and the cow seemed unwilling to give me much assistance.

I was sweating buckets, partly through the physical exertion of trying to get the calf out and partly because the day was warming up to a scorcher. Progress getting the calf delivered was slow, my early impressions of it being a big calf seemed correct, and I was certain that the calf would be stillborn when it was delivered, there seemed no sign of life whatsoever.

Jane appeared to see what was happening and to see if we all wanted a drink. It was the first time in all the years she had known me that she had observed me working as a vet, hands, and arms deep inside the cow and me getting increasingly covered in whatever came out of both openings of the back end of a cow. Helper Bob and I got the usual comments about we did not know the pains of childbirth, but I was fairly sure I knew what the cow standing in front of me was going through. Jane did hang around to watch proceedings as inch by inch we were making progress in delivering the calf. The calf ambulance was summoned, I had corrected the twist in delivery and first the front legs, then the head, the shoulders and the chest of the calf became visible. Yes, this calf was massive and still mum showed no desire to push whatsoever, all the effort was coming from me, and inside my overalls now it felt like I was having a sauna.

Jane was fascinated watching her first calving, phone camera ready to capture the moment the calf was delivered into this world. We were there, the large hips of the calf came gently through the cow's pelvis, back legs following and slipped gently into the wheelbarrow. We were finished, the calf was out but checking it as suspected showed no signs of life. Disappointing after so much effort and for mum who would have no calf to rear, and as previously said, she was a very maternal cow. Examining the calf led me to believe that the calf had died thirty-six/forty-eight hours ago. There was no sign of calving until a couple of hours previously, there was nothing else we could have done in the situation.

But again, very disappointing for all involved and especially for Jane who did not get to see a live calf delivered. This was certainly the biggest calf that had been delivered in this calving season at Bob's, it was massive. But that's nature, there was nothing more we could have done in the circumstances.

I just had to decide now what to do with the cow. Having been warned of her temperament at calving time, I decided the best we could do was to inject her with antibiotic and anti-inflammatories and return her back to the group of cows she had come from, hoping she would pass her afterbirth naturally by herself, and that we wouldn't have to handle her again. We let her back into the field and had that hard earned drink that Jane had come to enquire if we wanted. Very much appreciated in this heat before for me, stripping off and having a shower.

I kept a close eye on the cow and later that day she did pass her afterbirth, but I remained wary of her, every time I came to the field she would come up to the fence as if she knew there was something missing, her calf. But over the next few days she did settle down to become just another member of the herd.

The days got hotter, the grass grew less and less and at the end of the week it was time to move the cows onto fresh pasture, or more truthfully another large field that had slightly more grass on it than the one they were on. They were queuing by the gate as if they knew this was the day they should move, and with the help of Pete and helper Bob, they were soon moved across the track and onto this new pasture and as they settled down in their we were able to move the hay racks and creep feeder over from one field into this one. They seemed settled and had plenty of preserved forage to see them over the coming weekend.

This day was predicted to be the hottest day of the year so far with temperatures supposed to be going into the mid-thirties Centigrade. Thankfully today there was a slight breeze which made life a lot more comfortable. I had taken myself into Newport to explore before lunch, taking myself along the old Newport canal and into town. It was lovely to see the Mayflies hovering over the water, the young coots, moorhens, and cygnets exploring the waterway between the lily pads. Elder in blossom, English nature near mid-summer at its best.

Jane had taken her metal detector with her to the farm and hoped to spend a lot of time exploring the fields looking for that unexpected surprise lurking beneath the soil. I had promised her that afternoon that I would go out with her and help dig the buried treasure when she found it. We went out on the field that the cows had been moved from earlier and it was not long before her machine was making encouraging noises. But the trouble was that the soil was now baked so hard that I could not even make an impression on the soil to find what was causing the bleep. We explored elsewhere but every time she asked me to dig, it was hopeless, I needed a pickaxe.

We gave up and decided another day we would go onto the peat soils and see if we had better success. She was going to return to the house, I said I could hear a lot of bellowing of cattle, something, somewhere must be up. I would go and investigate. Not being a cowgirl, she was fascinated that just by listening to our surrounds that I could tell something was amiss.

I set off towards the field where Bob's cows were, not that this was where the noise appeared to be coming from. I wandered around the cows, they all seemed quite settled but still I could sense something was not right. There was a copse between his and his neighbours land and to me that was where the noise was coming from, so next I went over to check through this, but still nothing. I had looked everywhere I could think of but had found nothing. I had to give up and set off back towards the house across the field we had been detecting in.

There were many thistles in this paddock, I had started cutting down some of them with my small scythe but on the slopes, there were huge clumps of the weed. I was walking through them when I noticed something black. Lying hidden was a calf, left behind by mum when we had moved them earlier in the day. He got unsteadily to his legs, and it became obvious that on this sweltering day and without mum to suckle from that he was getting dehydrated. I tried to stir him quietly towards the gate the cows and calves had gone through earlier, while ringing Jane and getting her to find the key for the padlock on the gate, come down the track and open the bate when I had the calf near it so it could re-join the rest of the herd, and mum.

I nearly had the calf where I wanted, Jane opened the gates between the fields. But now mum realised this was her calf and came charging towards the gate. Now Jane is not a cow person, she was not going to stand there with this big cow running towards her. I now had a cow and a calf in my field and running in the opposite direction I wanted them to do, the calf seemed suddenly to have regained his energy. They did eventually stop, and slowly but surely, I was able to direct them back towards the gateway and field that I wanted them to be in. Jane had closed the gate again to stop the other cows following, not that they had wanted to, they had been starring at this field for the past two days and were not going to leave it if they did not have to. At the appropriate moment, she opened the gate, cow and calf were re-united with the rest of the herd.

We closed the gate and then watched as calf started suckling vigorously from mum, if he was dehydrated, he would soon rectify the situation himself. But it would be another animal I would keep a close eye on over the next couple of days.

Jane and I wandered back towards the house and again she was fascinated that my intuition had told me that something was wrong, and that we had solved the problem. All was quiet, a later check would show all well with the calf. But I would keep a close eye on him for the rest of the time I was in charge. He was a busting bull calf, and it would turn out when Bob got home that this cow had calved on the quiet while I was in charge. She never showed any signs, nor did I see any afterbirth at any stage. I wondered why this calf had no ear tag yet, but all was well in the end, and it was nice that a cow had calved naturally without any problems.

It was time to light that barbeque on the patio that night and enjoy a couple of those steaks that Bob and Venessa had left us. And they were delicious, we had discovered that one of the local supermarket's ribeye's were excellent. These had come from there.

We had to deal with the bull that needed a casualty slaughter, he was lame and was not going to recover. It seemed a shame having fed him for a few days and him gaining faith that I was his buddy that I had to let him down, but in the long term it was the kindest thing for him. My helpers had not experienced this on-farm slaughter before, he was not fit to travel, and perhaps it is not the nicest thing to experience but it had to be done one Way or the other, hopefully this would be the only downside of my few days in charge.

I was having to come back to Telford every other day to look after my tomatoes, check any post and to take care of some elderflower champagne I was making. Bob's farm had contributed some of the elderflowers. It needed to ferment and later to be bottled to wait until Jane and I would drink it, chilled out of the fridge.

Little did I know then what an explosive brew this would be. We were sitting at home some days later when one evening a heard a bang, it sounded as if something had fallen on the floor somewhere in the house. On investigation I found nothing, a mystery. It was a couple of days later that I went into our front shed to find a distinct smell of elderflower, this is where I had put all the filled bottles, and then broken glass and champagne all over the shelves. Jane had suggested that I used some plastic bottles her fizzy water came in as well as used wine bottles. The pressure building up inside these had split them wide open. What a mess

I had to clear up and even some weeks later I was still finding shards of glass in the shed.

I had made a start on all those thistles but in the soaring temperatures and with a scythe with only a short handle it was hard work, and with some of these thistles being nearly as tall as me they often fell towards me and I was getting many tiny pricks in my fingers as I tried to chop them all down. My brother brought my mother out to the farm, he thought it would be nice for her top see a farm again after so many years, and he had managed to retrieve a long-handled scythe my father had which he had lent to a neighbour. Sharpened as well, there would now be no mercy for these weeds. For an hour a day or when I went to look around the cattle, armed with scythe, I was now making real progress in clearing them, but I knew it would be beyond my wildest dreams to clear them all before my duties were finished. But bit by bit I was making progress and in doing so, uncovering some lush grass, to be honest the only decent looking grass in these cow paddocks. But it was demanding work as the temperatures remained high, "mad dogs and Englishmen out in the midday sun"!

We would have to move the cows again from time to time, though with so little grass growth, how we needed rain, there seemed little point. We would be feeding them heavily with supplementary hay and silage in their racks. In the end I decided we would leave them on the peaty fields, it did retain any moisture left in the ground better, and it was not burning up like the rest of the farm. You could see this with the naked eye.

A bit of gardening now and again, watering Venessa's beautiful begonias, now exhibiting a wonderful show of colours, some beautiful roses (one gorgeous one with white flowers which had a pink tinge around the edge of all the petals). And the tomatoes in their greenhouse needed constant watering, especially with the thermometer in the greenhouse showing temperatures more than fifty degrees Centigrade most days.

The house was extremely comfortable, I was enjoying myself being a farmer again, and Jane was enjoying a change of scenery as well. The days were slipping by, and I was pleased to get messages from Italy of how much Bob and Venessa were enjoying the chance to relax. It made it even more worthwhile for me.

The days were slipping by. My days as a farmer, Jane as a farmer's wife would soon be ending. I enjoyed another couple of walks into Newport, keen to see how those young birds were fairing on the waterway. All this young life did seem to annoy the swans who sometimes were quite aggressive to me as a passer-by. I in future would give them a wide berth, I did not want to incur their wrath too much.

The sun beat down and we prayed for rain, though it would take a good downpour to soak into the baked ground. But none was forthcoming, even if the temperature did drop a little and a gentle breeze made the temperature more bearable. Jane hoped we could go out with her metal detector her again before we returned home so on our last but one day off, we went again but this time to the side of the farm that was peat. There were a few bare areas, so we tried these and eventually got the sounds she was looking for. There was definitely something there to dig for and after a few minutes we had a large, rusted object in her hand. She was convinced it was some ancient weaponry artifact, about five inches long and pointed. A fancy it was the end of a tine from a fore loader when muck carting. Who knows, but it is stored away for posterity.

It was our last night there together, Jane would return home the next day, I would spend one last night there by myself and then return the following afternoon after feeding. Bob and Venessa would return later that night, as it happened, somewhat later than expected with the airport delays especially at Manchester. It was lucky I did not stay there until their return; it would have been a late night. Jane and I decided we would have a barbeque, enjoying the early evening sunshine on the patio one last time. A nice bottle of Rioja and another enjoyable steak was a fitting tribute to our last night there together. One last bedtime and we were spoilt by the most wonderful sunset, it was near the summer solstice, and we were to see the most spectacular sky of our whole visit. It was worth staying by the window until the whole scene had finished with the sun finally disappearing below the horizon. On reflection, I think it was the best sunset I had seen the whole of the 2022 summer.

Jane departed the next morning; I was left at the farm by myself. Pete and I had a big tidying up session around the yards, in the sheds, wherever we felt the place could be tidied. I hoped Bob would be pleased with the farm he was going to come back to. The cattle looked well fed and were putting on condition, as we had hoped with the impending sale. The farm tidy, several thousand less thistles in the fields now. What we could not make happen was for the grass to grow and to make it rain. That situation did not really change the whole of the summer.

One last night in the house, a final day of feeding and when the evening one was done my days as a farmer had finished. I had really enjoyed the experience again after so many years. There had been a bit of vetting, a little bit of paperwork to do and notes to write for Bob on his return. I loaded the last of my things in the car, including the scythe. Those thistles that had survived my stay would live to flower and spread their seeds accordingly. Next year's crop!

It did seem like a return to my roots, from helping dad all those years ago when I was left in charge of his dairy farm while he and mum tried to take a break from all their hard work. A change from being a vet and a change now from retirement, but I think if asked then if I would like a little holding of my own and a few animals, the answer would be no, I, we liked to get away when we could without the commitment of having our own animals and having to get someone to look after them in our absence.

Over the coming days and weeks I would help Bob with his stock, when they needed moving, when some needed sorting out at times such as weaning and especially on that final day for the cows when we had to load them onto the lorries to take them up to Carlisle for his dispersal sale. A sad day for him after forty-five years of breeding of his pedigree herd but we all must stop sometime. I hope that I had made those final few days, weeks of his more bearable for him. We started playing golf together to give him some sort of relaxation away from those stressful last few days he had the herd with so much to do related to the sale.

I think somewhere in my retirement plan I had a wish to start playing golf again and it was now finally happening. I did go up to Carlisle to support him at the sale, stopping on the way the previous day to at last climb the 950 metres of Helvellyn, something else that had been on the wish list for a couple of years, but now another thing ticked off on my list.

It was now time to settle into retirement fully. Or would I?

INTO THE SUNSET:

SOMEWHERE IN MY memory was there not talk of a retirement party, a chance to say goodbye and thank you to so many of my loyal clients from over the years, as well as members of staff that because of Covid restrictions I had never had the chance to say my farewells to properly. Calling in on James Turnock one day for a coffee, he had remarked that as he had sold his dairy herd some months earlier before Covid, that he had very soon lost contact with his fellow dairy farmers and as he said, "You are very soon forgotten!"

I guess sadly that I was beginning to think the same. While restrictions on social gatherings were still in place because of the pandemic, then a party was impractical and improbable. It seemed like it was never going to happen and with that I was beginning to agree with James, and that if it did eventually take place then it would all fall a bit flat for me. Not the way I wanted to go out so was it better just to forget about it.

I had of course kept in contact with some of the staff and had needed to see and speak to a couple of them because of my involvement in the Avian Flu outbreak, essentially though working for APHA. I was doing so sub-contracted to Shropshire Farm Vets. Tia and I chatted from time to time, and she kept on saying that we would have my party but with the restrictions, she could not say when.

I was losing heart over it a little.

It would have been nearly a year after I had officially retired that she did get in touch and asking if I had any ideas what I would like to do, it looked like the pandemic was coming under some sort of control, restrictions would be lifted so it was possible that later in the summer we could do something, even if meant having a couple of events with restricted numbers.

"What would I like to do, did I have anything in mind"?

The honest answer to that was no and that I would have to think about it, she would too. It was difficult as I did not know what the Directors would want to spend on it, how many people would come and how many staff would be invited. On my visits to the office, each time there seemed more and more people that I did not recognise. I did not want the situation where all members of staff felt they should be invited which would restrict the number of farmers, and that then at my party I would not know half the people who were there. The other question would be what day of the week, after so long would people want to give up a weekend night or would we have to go for a weekday, then with the farming cycle, would that clash with silaging, haymaking, harvesting. It worried me that it could all be arranged and that not many people would be able to come, I would be disappointed.

I would put my mind to it, but obviously Tia had done more than that. I received an email from her saying what about going on the *Sabrina*. The Sabrina is a motorboat which can hold up to sixty people that sails up and down the Severn in Shrewsbury at various times of day. I did not know what sort of party Tia had in mind but for me this boat had incredibly happy memories. I had been on her once before and that had been on my wedding day five years previously, Jane and my special day. We had got married at Shrewsbury Castle, overlooking part of the loop of the river that all but surrounds the centre of the town. We were married by just gone three in the afternoon, we had the best part of four hours to kill before our small reception/wedding breakfast would be held in our favourite restaurant in town, *Renaissance*, for the fourteen special guests plus ourselves. We decided we would hire *Sabrina* for the afternoon, walking down from the castle to the boat to board and then spend a pleasant couple of hours on the river before we ate later. We could say goodbye to the rest of our guests in the pub opposite when we had disembarked from the boat then when the time came, walk back into town to the restaurant. We had been blessed with fine weather, a wonderful sunny summers afternoon, great company and a very happy day for the new wife and me.

Now to have the opportunity to have my retirement party on the boat as well, an opportunity I jumped at when Tia offered it to me. The only question was when and what time. It may have to be late afternoon on a Friday in July or August before they did their evening meal and trip for which they were fully booked up throughout the summer months.

Tia would get back to me with a date, we had a quick chat about those to invite to include staff and clients although numbers we would be unsure of. We had discussed as I left the invitees, not all may be able to come and there were a few other names that I had thought of that I would like to have come.

But the thought of being on the *Sabrina* again was enough for me to look forward to even if it was only going to be a short early evening adieu.

It was not long before Tia offered me a date, there had been a cancellation for July 2nd., we could have the boat on a Saturday evening from seven thirty for three hours.

"What did I think?"

"This was perfect, "I said, "It would be just the sort of send-off that I really wanted."

The rest was now up to Tia to arrange other than Jane and I sorting out what we wanted from the menu, and the choice of foods was far more than I was expecting. I eagerly anticipated the evening, hoping that I was going to have the sort of final send-off I wanted. I really appreciated all that Tia had done in arranging this, but she very kindly said that "for all I had done for the practice and for the profession over the years, it was no more than I deserved."

That would have been a lovely epitaph.

But briefly, I will jump ahead to the following weekend after my leaving do. I had been to Newport Show once in my life, a large and very popular agricultural show though with many other stands to interest all members of the general public. My brother had got

me a couple of tickets and again on another hot summers day Jane
and I set off to enjoy a day out there. I hoped I would bump into
a few of my old farm clients as well as meet up with some of the
vets from surrounding practices who would have a stand there.
It was just up the road from Bob and Venessa's, but they were
unsure whether or not they would be going. On such a glorious
day the whole town and surrounding area had decided to go so we
queued for some time to get in, but once there were able to enjoy
a particularly good show.

I did want to go around the cattle and sheep lines as I was
certain that I would bump into some old acquaintances exhibiting
their show animals. As well as the common breeds of cattle, there
were some of the rarer breeds as well, Highland cattle, Longhorns,
and others. I suppose experience had told me to look downwards
where cattle may have walked before you, Jane did not and it
was not long before she had some brown, warm and smelly stuff
oozing between her toes and over her sandals. Luckily, I bumped
into the husband of a girl I had worked with at a previous practice
who recognised me and very graciously got a bucket of water and
washed Jane's feet for her. The sun soon dried them. But walking
further through the lines we did meet old clients who had heard
of the party for me, good things and were pleased that I had been
given a good send off. And we did bump into Bob and Venessa and
shared a drink with them as well.

We had to leave early as we had been invited to an evening
wedding party later, the other side of Shrewsbury, be there for
seven thirty. We changed and set off, me being a little apprehensive
as we got there as to how much Jane would enjoy it as other than
the groom's parents, it was unlikely that she would know anyone
else there, and obviously they would have other guests and family
to deal with.

A marquis in the middle of a field, near a pond with some
wonderful oak trees surrounding it (some of whose boughs I was
later informed were used in the repair of York Minster). A beautiful
setting for what I was told had been a wonderful ceremony.

But I was right, there was nobody else we knew other than the main participants at a wedding, and they were busy having the photographs taken around the pond, a stage adorned with white flowers as a backdrop to those special pictures. We were told there was food but after a couple of hours and no sign of it we were getting hungry. At last, I was able to have a chat with Peter, the father of the groom who had been on the Sabrina the previous weekend. I took him for a walk, he looked like he needed a break from the wedding festivities, and we talked about the day, the oak trees, and about my leaving party which he and his wife had much enjoyed. We reminisced what a pleasant evening it had been, and he very kindly said that I would not be forgotten.

But back to the party and he then kindly queued for us to get us a pizza, the food that was promised. And then we did meet some of my past clients who were so pleased to see me and to say goodbye properly. And again, the wonderful things they said about me. They mentioned the leaving party and I was embarrassed that they may be offended that they had not been invited, but all they said was that they had heard through the grapevine that it had been a great evening and that they were pleased that I had been given a proper send-off.

A lovely day and evening to meet and say farewell to more clients, and it was a beautiful evening. A more than happy day for two people, and for me, as well as being able to participate in this special day, another chance to see people who I had enjoyed working with/for but never had got the chance to say farewell.

But back to the *Sabrina*, the night of my leaving party had finally arrived. I had found out that a couple of the farmers and their wives who I hoped would be invited were not able to come for one reason or another. One of them, Jim and Fiona had invited myself and Jane, Bob and Venessa over for a meal a few nights beforehand and as it was over twelve months since I had left, it was nice to reacquaint myself with their farm again, such a big enterprise and it was interesting to see how things had moved forward, even in such a short space of time. How they were using modern technology to make better use of that organic asset that came out of the back end of cows, being able to separate the nitrogen from the potash and phosphate components to manage better the fertilising of their land, something I have described earlier.

We had made our choices from the menu for the Sabrina, I knew Jane would not remember but I had them in my head. Tia had given instructions for us to be there by seven so the boat could leave on time from the quay at seven thirty. It transpired that we had got the boat for the whole evening. Tia had also asked me if I wanted to say a few words and I could promote my book, *"The Quiet Vet"* which had just been published. Of course, I would love to say a few words, my career crammed into a few short minutes.

We were going to be spoilt. Gone were the cloudy days that had preceded this special night for me, the sun was shining as we arrived in Shrewsbury to leave the car close to where our voyage was to begin. We walked over the Welsh Bridge, looking over to see the *Sabrina* waiting for us and a small crowd were waiting to board when we would be permitted on board. As we made our way along that familiar path towards the Armoury, I was pleased to see familiar faces from my working days, some that I had not expected to be their but was really pleased to see them. Faces I had not seen since I had left but who had given up their Saturday evening to join me in my swansong. One or two gifts were given to me as leaving presents, but I also had to introduce Jane to fresh faces she had not met before as well as those familiar to her.

I knew Siobhan and her partner could not make it, but it was lovely to see Charlotte there as well as Calin from the Tb testing team. At the appointed time we were permitted onto the boat, there was a seating plan so once we had found our tables, our seats, we were soon able to embark on our voyage. Our previous voyage on our wedding day had taken us downstream towards the English Bridge, under it towards the weir before turning and returning to the mooring. I wondered how many times we would have to do this to occupy the amount of time the boat was hired for.

There were just over thirty of us and as we set off, I was

worried that I had not seen Cristina and Alex from the team who had become more than good friends. We were all seated on the top deck of the boat, tables of four, me closest to where our captain was steering the boat. I realised soon after that they had sneaked on unnoticed by myself and were at the other end of the boat, I would catch up with them when I could. But for now, Jane and I had the company of Jill and Dan who had also accompanied us on our wedding day trip.

We did head towards the English Bridge then return, by which time our meal was starting to be served to us. Drinks on the house, well provided by my former employers this was looking to be a wonderful and memorable night. Would we turn around and head back the way we had just come? I did not know, and wondered when we went back to the mooring again whether we would just stay there until our time was up. But no, we had just stopped to let the chef off, his work was finished. Then we were back underway but now heading under the Welsh Bridge and continued upstream on that enormous loop of the Severn in Shrewsbury.

The meal was excellent, far better than I had expected from a small galley aboard a boat with limited time to prepare. Tasty food, good wine, and great company, this was turning into a very enjoyable evening, and still the sun shone as it started to dip towards a sunset. Despite the great company among devoted friends on our table, it was time for me to circulate amongst all my guests. Talk of what I was doing in retirement and of some of the good times we had spent together in my days as a vet in Shropshire. Some of these people had been with me since I first came to Shropshire, others had been clients in my first practice, and we had met up again in my last. Those that I had worked with, those for which I had worked.

What better way to spend an evening, and then we were blessed with seeing a kingfisher patrolling the banks of the river. Of course, the summer of 2022 had been dry, the river was low, and I wondered how far we would be able to navigate upstream before we ran out of water below us. Certainly, the sand banks dipping into the river were becoming more and more pronounced, it was time to turn around both because the river wouldn't let us go much further and because our time was running out.

It was time to say a few words. Alistair stood up and thanked me for my past services, adding that I had always put everyone else first before my own needs. That was a lovely thing to say, and with those few words, the floor was mine.

It was an emotional time for me, always known to be quiet, but with a mic and the peaceful surrounds of a summers night on the river I would be heard. If I had sort of prepared a speech, a few notes written on a scrap of paper, that was soon discarded, I could speak from my heart at what a pleasure it had been to work for these people over the past thirty plus years. They would never be forgotten, there would be many times when I would reflect on my career as a vet. Generous, friendly, it had been rewarding and a pleasure to service them over all those years, some I would now count as lifelong friends, others I would see when I could, even if as we envisaged, Jane and my future would not be in Shropshire. And of course, a special thanks to my employers, two of which were here, two who could not be, family or work duties. One could not attend an emergency call if you were stuck on a boat on the Severn!

Yes, I did mention the book, but only in as much as it was a dedication to the people I had served over all those years because without them, this career could not have happened. I hoped what I had said went down well, I was always a nervous speaker as to what I would say and hopefully without too many ums. It was time to talk to everybody again individually, circulate amongst my guests. The sun was now fast setting and soon we would be back at our mooring, the evening over and time to say our goodbyes.

The evening had been more than I had hoped for, a very generous tribute to my years as working as a vet and my time working for Shropshire Farm Vets. I was grateful for all the support both farmers, my fellow vets, my employers, and my other work colleagues had given me over my past years in the practice. But my memories went beyond that, to those times in Devon and Gloucestershire as well, to those times as a farmer's son and through my training. Happy memories through all those years and as we came slowly back to shore, back onto the hard banks of the River Severn, perhaps now was the fitting time to call it a day.

I would see all these people again I hoped, they had been part of my life for so long and with so many of those happy memories. It had been lovely to finish it all sharing the company of Dan and Jill, Cristina and Alex, Alistair and Tia, Peter and Julie, Charlotte, James, so many.

As we came to the end of our voyage, the captain of the *Sabrina*, steering the boat from just behind where I was sitting also wished me well in my retirement, and me to him to thank him and his crew for an unforgettable evening.

The company had been fantastic, food excellent, everybody said they had enjoyed a lovely evening, and it all had been in honour of me and my career. In the end I had managed to have my chance to say goodbye properly and it had taken place somewhere that I, Jane and I, already had so many happy memories of.

As with our wedding day, we had been spoilt by the weather, a glorious summers day and evening.

As we returned to shore, as darkness began to fall, then it really had been a fitting end to my career, "The Quiet Vet" into the sunset of his career.

Thank you to all who made it as it was.

The Quiet Vet.... into the sunset.

POSTSCRIPT:

MAY 2023:
It has been two years since I walked out of the office for the last time. Two years into retirement, though I have been through the office door a few times since then with doing some Tb testing for the practice, and keeping in touch. Those two years have been very busy, as they say when you finish, "How did I ever find time to work"!

Yes, I have kept my hand in a bit, especially spending a second winter carrying out Avian Flu work which has taken me to various parts of the country doing surveillance work. In that I have met more wonderful people, interesting folks carrying out those traditional rural pursuits like saddlery, farriery and even meeting one guy who in since past spare time helped to do up Spitfires, Hurricanes and Messerschmitt's. Fascinating tales they all have to tell and it has been interesting chatting to them.

A little bit of cattle work has kept my interest on that side, helping friends with the odd Tb test, the odd poorly cow or calf and of course, a few calvings. It would not have been many days ago that Bob rang me one Saturday night with a cow calving, a relief for him as he was going to Italy the following day for a ten day break. He could go, happy that everything that should have calved had. I arrived at dusk and when we had got the cow in from the field I examined her. There was no way this cow was going to calve then or for the next few hours. I told him to get on that plane and go, I would keep an eye on her for him. Daily visits to look at her and she was getting a bit fed up with my company, turning her out, bringing her back in again, and with frequent messages from Italy, "Has she calved yet"?

She was getting fed up, but finally some ten days later I arrived to check her, and she just turned and looked at me as if to say, "Rod, I need some help now."

She looked uncomfortable and so I got her into the crush yet again, and putting my hand inside her, yes, today was the day. I managed to get a nice live heifer calf from her and duly put her back in the shed, though after her asking for my help, she was now very possessive of her calf and not happy for human attention. I messaged Bob, "At last she had produced, but don't go into the pen by yourself"! He arrived back from Italy thirty six hours later so missing the dramas of the previous few days.

But in the end, a nice result for me to welcome him home with.

So, have I missed it. Yes, I do really enjoy those few days I now have working with cattle, it has been my whole life. No, I do not miss those early mornings, it is nice now to work when I want to, and saying that I no doubt will do a few days of Bird Flu next winter if required, the money earned will take me back to Africa. The Serengeti, Ngorongoro calls me from afar, somewhere else to tick off my bucket list.

Another Jurassic challenge just completed, twenty six miles of hard walking of which stubbornness and grit got me through to the finish line.

But just a footnote on a couple of things before I finish. I wish maybe that I had known I would enjoy writing in my latter years, if so I may have made notes on some of what I had seen over all those years as a vet.

Those triplets I delivered all those years ago, seventeen to be precise. If one of them last year finally succumbed to the rigors of wear and tear on a farm, suffering severely from arthritis, and having to be put to sleep, then the other two still live a happy life, one now retired and enjoying her days just eating grass, the other just having produced yet another calf. And both of them can stand proud in their field with some of their progeny sharing the grazing with them.

I had hoped that there would still be a future for the small dairy farmer like dad was all those years ago. But despite Brexit, we have decided to comply with some of their regulations still. Something under the long winded name of "Storing-silage-slurry-and agricultural fuel oil" regulations means that these small dairy units have to install greater storage capacity facilities for their slurry and drainage water off their cow yards, something that will be very expensive and that they may never recoup the return on their "investment". Sadly it will make the job uneconomic for them. The days of the small family dairy units that I grew up with are very sadly numbered. I hope it will not also be to the detriment of the countryside because many of these farmers really did look after their rural surrounds. A sad day.

I have written a little again about wellbeing and mental health issues in the rural and veterinary community. I hope that the support groups around continue to thrive, though it would be nice to think that their need would become less and less as we all become more aware of the issues people face.

But many thanks to Chris at Shropshire Rural Support for the help she gave me in finding out about their work, and also to Vetlife for the information that they have sent me in supporting the veterinary profession.

Also, many thanks to all who have helped, contributed, those who I have worked with, both vets, nurses and support staff. Without you all, life may have been somewhat dull!

Life as a farm vet has had its ups and downs, but on the whole it has been a wonderful career, enabling me to work with some wonderful people and in the English countryside I so much enjoy.

Happy days!!